Margo R. Wickersham

Gratitude
in the
Storm

*When
not dying
is enough
to keep
fighting*

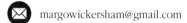 margowickersham@gmail.com

instagram.com/MargoWickersham

linkedin.com/in/MargoWickersham

facebook.com/MargoWickersham

twitter.com/MargoWickersham

tiktok.com/@MargoWickersham

bit.ly/MargoYoutube

Editorial direction by Phyllis Jask

Cover and text design by Brenda Hawkes

Printed in the United States of America

ISBN-13: 979-8-4399044-7-1

To my husband, Coleman Jennings, my children

Read Winter and Rachel Winter, and my friends and family

who have loved and supported me through my struggles and

shared in my triumphs.

Contents

Prologue

I was waiting for the oncologist to tell me if I still had cancer. As I sat there trying to avoid freaking out and catastrophizing, I got a call from the hospital saying my mother was dying and I needed to arrange hospice immediately. I felt the blood drain from my face and time slowed to a crawl.

I was in Houston, Texas, at MD Anderson, the number one cancer treatment hospital in the U.S. and one of the best in the world, and my mother was in Jacksonville, Florida—during the COVID-19 pandemic. This collision of simultaneous life or death events for me and my mother felt so overwhelming that I was paralyzed. In that moment, I couldn't think.

I reached for my husband's hand for comfort, but he wasn't there. I could only feel the pit in my stomach. Which do I think about right now? How could I possibly get through this moment, this hour, this day?

I felt unprepared for how to deal with these extreme stressors happening at the exact same time. Would I live or die? Will I get to see my mom before she dies? I had survived a lot of character-building challenges, but holy crap, this was scary, sad, potentially relieving, and happy all at the same time. Those are some extreme opposites! I felt alone, vulnerable, scared, and powerless.

I did the only thing I knew I could do in that moment. I inhaled deeply and steeled myself for what was to come. Channeling my inner Wonder Woman, I knew that I would handle whatever I had to, even if it seemed insurmountable.

And this felt impossibly insurmountable.

Introduction

This is the story of how I didn't die. I could have died, and if not for a second opinion, would have. I could have counted myself among the hundreds of thousands of people who died during the COVID-19 pandemic—the world's first pandemic in 100 years—but I don't. My story isn't really about death. Well, not my death, anyway. (Not gonna lie, there's some death in here.) It's not about COVID-19, either, although that's the landscape on which all this happened.

My story is part autobiography, part field guide. It's about life, living, and persevering through the unimaginable, surviving the unthinkable, and moving through misfortune by channeling my inner grit the whole way through in order to persevere all the way to the other side. Because, really, what choice do we have? We can give up, which is easiest and requires the least amount of effort. Or we can cling to a miniscule amount of gratitude to find something—anything—to appreciate in life to power us to take the next right step.

This is my story of how even during the violent storms in my life, a sliver of gratitude was all it took to keep me moving in the right direction. I'm not saying it was easy, and I'm not saying I didn't have help and care along the way. There were many, many times I wanted to give up—but I didn't. The journey isn't instant but it *is* possible. I'm living proof!

Here's something I learned: Life doesn't deliver challenges or problems to the human population evenly. However overwhelmed or burned out any of us feel, somewhere in the world there are always people suffering more but also people who have it easier than we do. Why does the unequal distribution of difficulties matter? It's not about comparative suffering; it's about collective strength. Accepting this truth frees us from the magnetic pull of self-pity. "Poor me" is easier to avoid when we realize we aren't alone in our human suffering. This is part of our common humanity and we each do the best we can to get through life and make it mean something.

When I'm feeling my most optimistic, I describe myself as fortunate to have had a bounty of opportunities to learn and develop character from. When I'm feeling a little (or a lot) less positive, I get overwhelmed and wander dangerously close to the "why me?" territory than I care to admit. Sometimes, I'll say to my husband, "I feel like I'm being greedy about character development. It's not fair for me to hog it all for myself and deny other people the opportunity to grow their character."

A decade ago, I restarted my career after a divorce and during a recession, after a 10-year hiatus raising kids. I spent the next 10 years as a working single mom, which any working single parent knows was really, really hard. I felt like I was trying to run through waist-deep wet concrete. I finally got my career and income back on track, although not as quickly as I expected.

Fast forward to 2020, the year that everyone wants to forget. I'm not kidding when I say 2020 was so full of challenges for me and my family that COVID-19 wasn't even in the top three. I battled an aggressive form of cancer and lost my mother and two other beloved family members in rapid succession. But I also pulled off a monumental opportunity for my employer the same year. Thank goodness we don't all suffer *all* the challenges all the time!

Like you, I've known many people who have fought difficult battles that come their way in life. Most fought as hard as they could. Some survived and others didn't. Life isn't fair. Some people found ways to go beyond survival and proceed to fully thrive. I'm one of them. It's so freeing to realize that either merely surviving or purposely thriving is choice that we can make. Our fate is not sealed, we do not need to feel doomed to a life of struggle for survival. Even during the messiest times, we *can* persevere and even thrive! I'm sharing what I've learned about getting through the outrageously difficult times, even when they last for years.

What can you control? Not the family or circumstances you were born into. Not the dynamics of your family of origin. Not your DNA. Not most of what happens to you growing up. The unlucky gene pool club has a variety of membership categories. You can be born into wealth but have a highly dysfunctional family of origin. Or you can be born into a modest or even impoverished circumstances but enjoy a warm, loving, and accepting family. Or you can be very unfortunate and born into poverty and dysfunction. Each of these scenarios earns you membership, but you'll attend different chapter meetings.

But you can control how you react to your circumstances. You can control what you do next. And what you think about and who you spend your time with. And collectively, these small decisions navigate the trajectory of your future. Whether our experiences are similar or not, our reactions will certainly vary. As someone who loves to learn from the wisdom of others as well as from my own experiences, I've discovered a few ways to weather the unexpected storms of life and created my own strategies that have helped me find joy when I thought there was none.

You are worthy of receiving love and living a happy and fulfilling life. Everyone is. If you are in one of the difficult phases of life that seems like it will never end, you may not know that prolonged struggle can trick your mind into thinking that this *is* your life, that this pattern *is* inescapable, and that hoping for better *is* going to lead to disappointment. These are all myths that your mind is tempting you to believe. Whatever your level of stress and exhaustion, I want you to know you are worthy of love, peace, and happiness. Even if you don't believe you are, I do and so do many others. (So try not to rain on our parade and stop us from believing in you and encouraging you, okay?)

My wish for you when reading this book is for you to feel hopeful, to know that any struggle you endure is temporary, and that choosing gratitude during dark times will help keep you in the right headspace so you can fight the good fight toward your end game. I wrote this book for you when you experience fatigue and want to find a way to keep going when your tank is empty. Whether it's pandemic fatigue (we all had that), parental fatigue, work fatigue, or juggling-all-the-hats-we-wear-fatigue, most of us reach a point where we are spent and need to double down. After receiving emotional and physical blows that seemed to never end, I discovered some ways to keep going even when I felt like giving up. I felt like giving up so many times, and it turns out that is *normal*. Phew! We humans are an extremely resilient species.

My goals in writing this book are sharing my story, providing hope for you if you're facing insurmountable obstacles, and sharing specific techniques you can use to persist, persevere, and flourish. It feels good to help others and this is one way that I can help. I encourage you to channel your collective strength to persevere and do more than just not die: Let's help each other *thrive*!

Trust me when I say I am not superhuman. I am, however, persistent. I've developed perseverance muscles from my experiences of facing what felt like insurmountable obstacles with sheer determination and grit. Sometimes, life just gets really, really messy and overwhelming. But every single time it did, I got back up. Sometimes I only barely got back up and it wasn't pretty, but I did it anyway. It's the getting up, not the falling down, that really matters.

How many times does a fighter have to get back up? As many times as it takes. Sometimes that is just one more. Other times, it's many more. I've learned that getting back up doesn't require that I *feel* like getting up. I can *feel* like giving up all I want. I can even take some time to pause and sulk before getting back up. But persisting, *whether you feel like it or not*, is the secret to success, however you define it. Because relentless perseverance— powered by a razor thin slice of gratitude—is what gets us through the punches that life throws at us so we can get to enjoying the happy stuff that helps us thrive.

PART 1:

Diagnosis

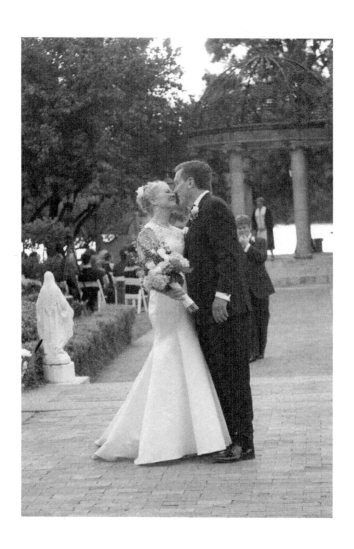

Chapter 1:
2019: Happy and Oblivious

Life was finally going well! My husband Coleman and I had just celebrated our third year of marriage and were blissfully happy. We enjoyed walking our two dogs every morning and working from home at jobs we both liked. We'd purchased our home in 2018 and were enjoying life in our new neighborhood. My kids were both in college and doing well. At long last, we had smooth sailing!

Adjusting to both kids out of my nest was a challenge, but I busied myself with work and embraced having the house to just my husband and me. One of the morning rituals that helped me start my day right, besides two cups of stout coffee with a splash of cream and one stevia, was to sit quietly and write at least 10 things I felt grateful for. I'd learned that focusing on gratitude releases happy hormones and relaxes our nervous systems. It sets our minds and bodies up for contentment and productivity. Of all the morning habits I've tried, I like this one best.

After journaling, I liked to do some stretching, but that didn't always happen. You know, life would get in the way. That May, I had started working for a start-up company that provided health care plans to self-employed people and I was busier than ever. I really enjoyed the people and the work we were doing. This was one of those sporadic times where both work and my personal life were great. It hadn't always been that way. Rarely do all the life cylinders fire in unison but in fall 2019, they were doing just that.

With more than 30 years' experience (that I'm admitting) in the business world—many working with start-ups—my instincts for knowing when the founders are truly caring people were well-honed. The company owners respected my insights and listened to my ideas. They were smart and exhibited a highly developed emotional quotient. Again, a rare quality to find at work, in my experience. The father-and-son team who created this company, Dave and Jackson, were uniquely caring, smart, and service-oriented leaders who were passionate about making a difference in the lives of people. Working for Clarity Benefits gave me a sense of purpose that doesn't come along in every job. I felt very fortunate to work with people I respected, and be doing work that made a difference in people's lives.

Plus, I *loved* working from home! Remember, this is 2019 when people went to offices every day from 8–5 and sat in traffic twice a day whether they liked it or not. I had just departed company with such a schedule, which also happened to be an incredibly toxic environment. I was grateful for this new job, its far less toxic environment, and to be providing a service that people needed. It all felt great!

Working from home has so many benefits, but social interaction was not among them. As an extrovert, I needed more socializing than was naturally built into my work week. (Now, nothing against introverts here. Some of the best salespeople I've ever hired were introverts. I deeply respect them and believe they are undervalued in our culture. They are great listeners and that is a superpower for selling!) My husband could always tell if I needed some "people time" and would encourage me to schedule time with a friend or colleague. A week of seeing no one outside of my house was too much. Going to an office every day 8–5 was also too much. I much prefer the former.

I was feeling really good about my work accomplishments. My job was to contact companies that hired thousands of contract workers—or 1099s—and create a partnership with them so we could offer our health care plans to their workers. I had found early success by landing a very large company as my first big account. EliteEdge was a real estate brokerage that had 22,000 real estate agents working as 1099s and the founder and CEO, John Whitaker, had promised a health care solution for agents. Clarity was the solution and we knew we had an incredible, albeit somewhat daunting, opportunity.

Clarity offered a health care plan that was less expensive than most health insurance plans available through the federal government's Affordable Care Act (ACA, or "Obamacare" as it's widely known) plans. Because health insurance plans traditionally have been delivered through employer-sponsored group plans, self-employed people like real estate agents did not have access to the "good" plans. Our company founders had discovered a way to offer plans that saved many agents a lot of money and provided better care than was available through the government site. Real estate agents were very excited about having better options that could save them money.

We built a website that encouraged agents to book a call with our licensed health insurance consultants. We had five consultants who took the calls and three managers who could jump in if the demand was high. It was and we all jumped in. I was one of the managers, along with the two co-founders. We all had full schedules with booked calls. It was a dream scenario!

The opportunity was enormous for our little start-up and we were energized by our excitement. We had worked around the clock preparing for the launch, but had made some missteps and were working through the troubleshooting. There was stress, but the outlook was good and the opportunity was terrific.

***

This was my first fall with both my kids in college and I could not wait to have them home for Thanksgiving! I texted them to find out what they wanted me to cook for Thanksgiving dinner and planned everything out. I love planning special occasions, especially when I get to see my kids! My son likes dark meat, mashed potatoes, and creamed corn. My daughter likes white meat, homemade dressing, and green beans. We all love dessert and I decided to have both pumpkin and pecan pies. Whether I made it or not was not the point. Some years I did, some years I didn't; it all depended on how much time I had. When I was a stay-at-home mom, I made everything myself. When I was a single working mom, I made very few homemade treats—and learned that HEB makes a damn good pie.

As we had in the past two years, we invited my husband's parents to join us. They were in their 80s and my father-in-law used a walker and was moving pretty slowly. We were grateful that our house had one story and had only one step up for him at the front door. CA and Lola were so small, and I mention this because their son, my husband Coleman, is 6'4" and we just can't figure where this height came from. If he hadn't resembled his parents, we might have thought the hospital gave them the wrong baby!

My mother-in-law, Lola, is a very caring, smart, and hard-working woman. She cooked everything from scratch. Like *scratch* scratch. She made her own tomato sauce from actual organic tomatoes, nothing from a can. She worked very hard to prepare healthy meals for herself and her husband because they were pre-diabetic. Loads of fresh fruit and vegetables! Lola was used to accommodating a wide variety of nutritional needs and was a very good cook. She had a way of making recipes not only more healthy but also more delicious.

Proud mama moment alert: My kids are very considerate of others and thoughtfully engaged in conversations with their step-grandparents. They were polite, attentive, and loving. By this time, they had only one grandparent alive—my mother, and she was in an assisted living facility in Jacksonville, Florida—so this was like a bonus inning of grandparents for them.

Rachel and Read helped me get everything ready and set the table. It was a beautiful table, which was more than a nod to my own grandmother, who always set "a beautiful table." I took a picture before everyone sat down and thought of my beloved grandmother fondly and lovingly. I relished (pun intended!) the time together with these three generations.

Our conversation was lively, and everyone enjoyed the dishes I'd made. Or at least was polite enough not to point out my shortcuts. At one point, Lola commented on how tasty the cranberry sauce was and asked how I prepared it. I answered, "I asked Read to open the can." We all nearly died laughing! Lola probably never served anything canned and I made no apologies for serving canned cranberry sauce to my family. I mean, at least I bought the kind with cranberry-looking orbs and not the kind that was shaped like a can, complete with the ridges! It was a fabulous and hilarious moment and we all enjoyed Thanksgiving together.

Some holiday memories stand out over others and Thanksgiving 2019 stood out for me. This was an especially warm and enjoyable day. I had my family together and we enjoyed each other immensely. Overall, November 2019 was a busy month with family visiting, my kids home from college, and me working hard at my new job. Maybe this holiday memory stands out more than others because it was the last multi-generational family gathering before worldwide and my own personal hell broke loose.

Chapter 2:
Playing the Grateful Game

Things in my life haven't always been as rosy as they were in Fall 2019. Which is why it felt natural to appreciate the smooth sailing. I think that's a common experience. It's hard to appreciate something we've always had. Gratitude comes easier after we've survived loss and begun to recover and feel better.

Life delivered some extremely tough blows to my children and me for several years before 2019. My kids talked about "our family curse." They saw disappointment after disappointment and experienced years of difficulty and struggle. I was determined to show them gratitude and perseverance.

Back in the dark ages—1989—when I endured my first divorce and consequently switched careers, I developed a coping skill for getting through hard times. I would vent to my friends and play what I called the "Grateful Game." I realized that thinking about something—anything—that made me feel grateful had the pleasant result of lifting my mood. So, when I felt discouraged, I'd talk it out with my friends and play the Grateful Game. What can I find to feel grateful for? I had a home to live in and keep me safe. I had friends who loved and supported me. I lived in Tampa, Florida, where I could see dolphins almost any day of the week! It was an inexpensive form of cognitive behavior modification, and served me well during some dark times.

The years spanning 2009–2015 were the most challenging ones I faced as a parent. We suffered a lot of trauma and loss. I was hell-bent on turning our lives around and providing years of more ease, more abundance, more happiness. It took longer than I'd hoped, but we did it, step by laborious step. The contrast of the difficult and even nightmarish times compared to how well life was going in fall 2019 made it easy to feel grateful, considering what we'd endured and overcome.

***

One evening in 2009, when my son was eight years old, he was in tears because he didn't understand why his father kept asking him the same question over and over again. That question was, "Do you love me, Read?" My husband at that time, Mark, was lying on the floor in our living room—drunk. His drinking had increased dramatically in the past few years and I was deeply concerned. I'd begun attending Al-Anon meetings to help me deal with it and had learned that the time to tell kids that a parent has the disease of alcoholism is when they notice strange behaviors caused by drinking. Once a child realizes that their parent is acting odd, it's helpful for an adult to identify the condition because if that doesn't happen, the child will internalize and blame themselves.

I took my son up to my six-year-old daughter's bedroom where she was playing and sat them down together on the bed, with my arm around them on either side and explained, "The reason your dad is lying on the floor asking you over and over if you love him, even though you kept answering that you did, is that he is drunk from too much beer. The reason he's been acting like this a lot is because he is an alcoholic. It's a disease and he doesn't currently have control over when or how much he drinks."

Boy, this is not something you want to have to tell your kids! They were so young. But I had to name it, now that one of them noticed the drunk behavior, or risk them thinking something was wrong with them. No way I was letting my children blame themselves for their father's drinking! They didn't really understand. The struggles we went through for the next decade were unfortunately numerous.

My kids' father never got sober. He lost his job and was out of work for a year and a half. I filed for divorce and we had to sell our house because we couldn't make the payments without his income. This was 2010, the very

bottom of the real estate market. We lost money on what was my dream
house. But as I like to say, "That was my dream house, but my nightmare
marriage." My life was beyond messy.

We moved from a beautiful home with a pool and view of the hills to
renting a funky old bungalow with a view of our neighbor's rickety garage
and old chicken coop—and not the cool urban chicken farmer kind, either.
It was a bit of a step down. I tried to make the best of the situation. At
least we could walk to the kids' school, only three blocks away. Also, we
could walk to the cafes and shops in Hyde Park about the same distance
in another direction. I was able to finally fulfil one of my life-long goals
of sending my kids to the corner store to buy butter and brown sugar to
make chocolate chip cookies. We managed to find fun and gratitude in an
otherwise dismal situation.

I scrambled all my resources to look for a job, but this was during the
Great Recession and I'd been out of the workforce for 10 years while I
raised kids. I joined LinkedIn, resurrected every professional contact I
could find, and updated my résumé. I finally landed an entry-level job as
a marketing assistant for a software company. It sucked to have once been
an executive at Dell and have to start over at the bottom, but I *had* to do
something to put food on the table. I did get a few bucks of child support,
but that didn't cover rent and there's no alimony in Texas.

One of the toughest things about this time in our lives was the phone call
I received from my son the afternoon of my first day of work. He was in
tears and said, "I want *you* to pick me up from school, not a baby sitter!"
As tears filled my own eyes, I answered him, "I know, Read. Me too. This is
how it is right now for us and it won't be like this forever. I don't know for
how long, but I do know we'll get through this." I felt so sad and deflated. I
wanted to hop in my minivan and get home to hold him and my daughter
for as long as they would let me. But, I was employed as a contractor and
paid hourly. I would not get paid if I left. I was so mad at my ex-husband
for putting us in this position, all because he couldn't put the bottle down!

I struggled to find compassion for my children's father. Al-Anon provided
me with a lot of support, although I must admit, I never quite achieved the

goal of feeling compassion for my "qualifier," as my ex was referred to in Al-Anon. I felt extremely angry and annoyed that he kept making terrible choices that impacted our kids and me so badly.

He'd gone to rehab in summer 2010 at a fancy facility in the hill country that his mother paid for. He was sober for about two months. Then he began dating a woman who started drinking her wine as she got her kids ready for school in the morning—a match made in hell.

I dipped into savings to take his ass back to court to make him blow into a breathalyzer when he came to pick up the kids. It's no fun at all to look for ways to protect your kids from their other parent. Even though my kids' father had no intention of hurting our children, his addiction was in charge of his decisions—and they were often terrible, like when he would show up drunk when he came to get the kids for his weekend. Yeah, it happened. Many times. And he did not get the kids when he showed up drunk.

He fought it, but the law was on my kids' side and we prevailed. Alcoholics will often try to blame others for holding them accountable for their sorry behavior. My ex was very unhappy about this new condition and guess what? He failed many times and couldn't have his own kids for an evening or weekend. It was beyond sad. But I had—and have—zero remorse and zero regrets for protecting my children.

Alcoholism is fatal if not treated. Mark's condition worsened. He got a third divorce, sold their house, lost his job, and squandered the inheritance his parents left him. He drank even more, which affected his relationships with our children. Our daughter stopped staying the night at his apartment. Once, during an out of town tennis tournament, our son had to drive his unconscious father to the hospital.

The hardest thing I ever had to tell my kids was that their father died. It's such a terrible story. One Saturday in late October 2015, the University of Texas Longhorns were playing football and my son, who was now 16, loved watching the games and talking with his dad about them. He began texting his dad after kickoff and didn't hear back from him. Read called his dad and it went to voicemail. Mark was a die-hard Horns fan. I used to say he put the fanatic back in fan. Not responding to a message from his son about the Longhorns was out of character. After no response for a couple of hours I knew he was either passed out (but he would have been at least quasi-awake for a Horns game), in a hospital, or dead.

I called Mark's brother Steve with my concern and he was worried, too. He couldn't reach Mark either. Steve called the apartment manager for the community where Mark lived to explore the option of getting a well check. Steve also called the police to see if they would check on him. Both options took a long time, since it wasn't a top priority. The day drew on with still no response from Mark. Steve and I texted and spoke on and off all day, trying to figure out what was going on. Read said he could drive over there to check on his dad, but he didn't, thankfully.

The police finally arrived in the evening and agreed to call to update me. Meanwhile, Coleman and I had tickets to see a flamenco band perform, and in between phone calls with Steve, we sat in the audience trying to enjoy the music. But I wasn't really there. Why wasn't I getting a callback from the police? I called the police after the performance to check on things and was told, "They are still on the *scene.*" The scene?! What the hell? I called Steve to see if he knew anything and we agreed that Coleman and I should drive over to Mark's place. It was late, after 10:00 pm now.

As we pulled up to the parking lot of Mark's apartment, I saw the homicide truck. I felt my heart drop into my stomach. As if watching myself from outside my body, Coleman and I entered the parking garage where the police cars were, worried about what we would find. We were greeted by a homicide detective wearing coverings on his head and his shoes. I heard myself say, "I'm looking for Mark Winter." The detective said, "Mr. Winter is deceased." Oh, my God. My worst fear—the worst possible outcome—was true! Expletives! Expletives! Expletives! The coroner hadn't arrived and they could not determine cause of death. What?

The detective asked me who I was, the nature of my relationship with Mark, etc., and I realized that of course I would be a suspect, because this was considered a homicide at this point. He asked if I would stay and be willing to talk with another detective in a few minutes. After agreeing, we went back to Coleman's car. Walking down the stairs with the news that the father of my children was dead felt like a lead suit that I had suddenly put on. I felt stiff, weird, and almost out of my body. And I'm going to be interviewed as a potential suspect? Not that I hadn't in my darkest hours occasionally fantasied about pushing him off the balcony when he passed out in front of the kids, but this was real and it conjured the most conflicting human emotions I'd ever felt.

Coleman and I sat in the car in disbelief. I said to him, "How am I going to tell my children their father is dead? That's the worst news ever!" Coleman was my boyfriend at this point and I told him how much I appreciated him being there with me for this dark, dark crisis. He's got one of the highest emotional quotients of anyone I know, so he was amazingly supportive in helping me work out what I would say to my kids. I knew I needed to be direct.

The detective who interviewed me seemed very nice but some of the answers she gave to my questions were perplexing. How did he die? "We don't know yet. It's hard to tell from the position he's in." What position? "Slumped over like this," she curved her body forward and to one side. That didn't make any sense. How could he be in that position? Wouldn't he have fallen out of the chair, if he'd been sitting? "When did he die?" I asked. "We won't know until the coroner gets here and they are out on another case." I knew, somehow, he'd died from alcohol abuse, but specifically how or when, I didn't know. But I assumed sometime that day.

She asked me if I had been arguing with Mark and other questions aimed at uncovering if I had motive. Certainly I would have had more motive when I was still married to him and had there still been any money left. As the second of his three ex-wives and the mother of his only children, I had no motive other than sheer exhaustion from raising children without his help and dealing with the impact of his alcoholism on our lives. I *so* didn't want to have to tell my children this news. Actually, I felt a new level of anger at this man for making me have to do this!

The detectives let me go and Coleman and I made our way back to my apartment. I walked in and said to my children, "Please come over to the table. I need to talk with you." I took Read's hand with my left hand and Rachel's hand with my right and said, "Your father has died. I am so, very sorry." Read threw his head back and shouted, "Noooooo!" Rachel, who was 14, appeared outwardly calm. My two kids have very different personalities and I knew they'd react and process differently.

My next words were, "We will each grieve in our own way and there is no one right way to grieve. We will get through this. I am here for you and we will be okay." Then I ushered them to the sofa so I could hug them both at the same time. We sat together for a long time. Read said, "I *knew* I should have gone over there to check on him!" I explained that he couldn't have done anything, that their dad's death was not in any way their responsibility and it is also very, very sad.

What none of us knew yet was that Mark had died in his car three days before, after pulling in from a midnight run to buy some more alcohol. When I learned that, I was so very grateful that my son had not been the one to find him. That was a silver lining in this extremely dark and shitty cloud.

Even in that dark hour I was able to channel something—anything—to be grateful for, a remnant of that skill I began developing in the 1980s that, along with others, came to my rescue many times in my life. The Grateful Game had ushered me through many troubling and challenging chapters. No matter how small the thing is that you can find to appreciate, gratitude for that one thing gives you just a little bit of umph to keep going. And that is all we need. A tiny, even microscopic sliver is enough to not die.

Fast forward to 2019. With this emotional and financial devastation behind me, I was thrilled to have a regular life! My family relationships were strong. We were no longer renters, dependent on the whims of a landlord's decisions to sell. Both my kids had graduated high school and were attending college. I was now happily married to Coleman. I had a great job that meant a lot to me. I felt extremely grateful, and dare I say even joyful!

Chapter 3:
Bad News

Three days after that lovely Thanksgiving in 2019, I noticed my urine was a deep rose color. That was new. I'd never had oddly colored urine. Post-asparagus consumption smelly, yes, Claret or Syrah-colored, never. By late afternoon, my urine was back to a normal color. Then the same thing happened the next day. That's not right. Concerned, I wondered what could cause this and did the only natural thing, which was to Google it. At 57, I knew this wasn't related to a menstrual cycle, so I took a sample to the lab. When the lab called to tell me the "good news," there was no bacteria in my urine, my heart sunk. According to Google, the other likely causes of blood in urine were kidney stones and bladder cancer. Scary. I know, never Google your symptoms, but I did anyway and decided getting more information was smart.

By this time in my life, I had developed my skills for coping with scary unknowns and told myself to quit worrying. If there's nothing to worry about, then any worrying would be needless and unhealthy. If it were something to worry about, I knew I'd have plenty of time to worry about it later. This strategy had served me very well to get through many difficult and frightening situations, helping me avoid useless and catastrophic worry. That doesn't mean it has been easy to do. And it also doesn't mean there wouldn't be times that warranted worry.

I called my OB/GYN nurse to ask what I should do. The nurse recommended "keeping an eye on it." I thought, "Nope. I'm not doing that. I'm going to a urologist as quickly as I can get an appointment," which turned out to be more than two weeks away on December 17.

Keeping my head down, I continued to work hard and long hours to lead my company through the challenging launch during the holidays and tried not to think about what could have caused the hematuria—that's med-speak for blood in your urine.

One Friday evening in late November, Coleman and I were grabbing a quick and relaxing dinner on the patio of our favorite Greek café when I got a call about my mother from her assisted living facility. The facility director said her blood pressure was extremely high, she was lethargic, and she needed to go to the hospital but was refusing. My heart sank. This wasn't the first time I'd received a call like this. My mother's mental and physical health had been declining for a couple of years. Anyone who's experienced the slow decline of a parent or loved one struggling with Alzheimer's, dementia, or any other debilitating disease knows how upsetting and draining the experience is. It's difficult to see them in pain and struggling, and it's disorienting and sad to see them as mere shells of their former selves.

***

Known as the "long goodbye," the terrible journey of dementia is painful for everyone involved. And yet, we want to make the most of the time left with our loved ones. It's one of the clearer examples of experiencing conflicting emotions at the same time. I felt so sad that my mother's mental faculties were declining, and I also felt appreciation for each moment of love and laughter that we experienced. At the same time. Sad and grateful simultaneously.

This began another very stressful chapter with the assisted living facility telling me that my mother required more care than they could provide. I lived in Austin, Texas, my mother lived in Jacksonville, Florida. I had a demanding job and was trying not to focus on my own health scare. How would I find time to shop for a nursing home too?

I scrambled and contacted the attorney who'd helped with my mother's affairs three years earlier and found a facility to check out. That first weekend of December 2019, I flew to Jacksonville to surprise my mother and take her on a tour of the nursing home. My mother was no longer able to manage keeping her phone charged or even answer it, so my visit was a surprise to her.

I found her sitting in the common room watching TV, wearing her fuchsia blouse with her long white hair pulled into a neat ponytail. She looked lovely. Even as an 83-year-old woman, she was still an elegant beauty. My mother was so happy to see me! Several other residents sat around as well and were happy for her that she had a visitor. We hugged and laughed. Because my mother had complained about the assisted living place, I explained that I had a new place for us to tour as a potential home for her.

I took her to visit Miller Rehabilitation and Hospital and toured the dining area, activity areas, and residential rooms. I had arranged for a mental evaluation for my mother to benchmark where she was cognitively and to create a plan of care for her. When the worker asked what city she lived in, my mother answered, "I couldn't tell you." My heart sank again. Although my mother could be lucid and carry on somewhat of a conversation, the other answers confirmed that she needed to be in a nursing home with memory care options. And this one accepted Medicaid.

Our smart, educated, and savvy mother had done everything she knew to do to prepare for her own retirement. It was hard for her to put my father (and not herself) through law school, spend 20 years raising kids, and get divorced at age 45 with minimal child support for my little brother. My sister and I were 18 and 19, so we were not considered a legal or financial obligation in their divorce.

Disciplined and determined, my mother saved and invested as much money as possible. But she was working with some serious financial handicaps. Her divorce was in 1981, so she got the worst of all deals: a little bit of money from equity in the house, just enough to buy a little condo for her and my brother. She received no alimony, since she'd recently earned an MBA and had "six-figure earning potential." Only the reality at that time was that a middle-aged woman starting her career in 1980 with no business experience did not in fact, enjoy the same opportunities that a man did. Things have improved so much in the past 40 years, but at that time things really sucked for her.

After years of severe financial difficulties, she declared bankruptcy. After the Great Recession, she lost the house she'd purchased after her divorce. She'd lived there 30 years and moved into a very small first-floor apartment nearby. By the time she was diagnosed with dementia and moved to assisted living, her savings had dwindled to around $70,000 and she was only receiving about $1,000 a month in social security.

Staying home to raise kids means you take yourself out of the social security pool for many years, which means you get a lot less. Being a divorced former stay-at-home-mom is a double whammy on top of that, since you don't get the shared household income from your spouse's social security. I know of women my mother's exact age who were also educated and stayed home to raise kids and remained married. They had literally 10 times the income my mother did because of all of those factors. Incredibly unfair for my mom and so many others.

To qualify for government aid, my mother needed to not have saved any money. We hired an attorney who specializes in helping families navigate the legal and financial waters for senior citizens and their families. The lawyer helped us spend our mother's life savings on things acceptable to the government, like pre-paying for final arrangements like a funeral and burial, among other items. Once the balance was lower, she "gifted" the money to me, her executor, with the understanding that I wouldn't spend this money. It was there if we needed it for her and if there was any left left upon her passing, it would be split among us three kids. The goal was to drain the accounts to less than $2,000, so we could qualify her for Medicaid.

Once on Medicaid, she would have access to assisted living facilities that accepted patients with it. The list of places that did was short and the waiting lists were long. It is not a good situation to be in. However, this attorney did succeed in helping us achieve that goal and even helped us find a place nearby. Mom would have to share a room with another woman, but at least we could get her in.

My mother lived there for a couple of years and her dementia seemed to stabilize. She could get around with a walker and even make it out for some shopping. I made quick trips to Jacksonville to see her when I could and my sister would visit her pretty regularly, as would our brother when he could get back to Jacksonville.

After this evaluation, I took my mother to the dining room to enjoy some dinner. They had vanilla ice cream, which Mom *loved*. While my mother enjoyed that treat, I drove to her assisted living home to begin loading her belongings so she could move into Miller Rehab. Some workers had kindly packed my mother's things. Some of her clothes were in packed into cardboard boxes with photos of women wearing adult diapers. "Ugh," I thought to myself, "this is what the life of my intelligent, elegant, and feisty mother had become." I saw myself going through the motions and felt like I was watching someone else. It was like a sad movie. I tried to fight back tears, but they won. I cried as I packed my mother's few belongings. Even the antique dough bowl that her grandmother had used to make bread and was so important to my mother was included in this move. It was so sad. She had been such a force, up to and including negatives to go with the positives. She and I had had a complicated mother-daughter dynamic throughout my life, so I chose to focus on the many positives in that relationship instead of the multitude of negatives that lived in my memory.

As I packed the rest of her photos, knick-knacks, and toiletries, I thought to myself, "I feel like I'm moving my third child into a new dorm room"— complete with a roommate, a little dorm fridge, a small TV, a couple of suitcases of clothes, and some personal items that all fit into a single car. Her roommate even had a poster of her heartthrob—Elvis Presley! Remember, this is 2020 at an assisted living facility with mostly elderly residents. And yes, it was the younger, slimmer Elvis, not the flashy and overweight Elvis of his later years. You're welcome for the visuals!

I remembered when my mom helped move me into Morrison dorm at the University of North Carolina in fall 1981. How could almost 40 years have gone by? I'd moved my own children into their dorm rooms. Now I was moving my mother into a senior living dorm room. It's not nearly as much fun, and it is sad in the worst way.

I checked on my mother in the dining room when I returned to Miller Rehab. She was still sitting in her chair listening to another resident talk, so

I quickly unloaded my mom's now tiny life and moved her into her new "dorm room," with her bed-bound roommate. I tried not to think about my own cancer worry and my upcoming appointment with the urologist. I wanted so badly to talk with my mom about my concerns and receive her love and encouragement. But I knew that she wouldn't understand and that would only worry and upset her.

When my mind wandered into worrying, I practiced some self-compassion and gently reminded myself to stay in the moment. Mindfulness was and still is something I continue to cultivate. Like all the best coping skills, it's a journey to develop them. This helped me refocus my attention to be present and enjoy the time with my mother, even as the task of moving her was difficult.

My sister Karen lived in Jacksonville and struggled with severe and rapidly cycling bipolar disorder. She did what she could do to help our mom, which included visiting her at the assisted living facility. Karen would bring our mother her favorite treats: Diet Coke and M&M's. My sister would send me pictures of their visits and I was so grateful she could and did see our mother frequently, especially because I lived in Texas and our brother lived in Virginia.

However, counting on my sister to show up and help me move our mother was not in the cards. Although Karen's intentions were good and I knew she loved our mother, her mental health issues kept her from being reliable. She was unable to help me move Mom's things, but she joined me for a Dollar Tree run to buy some Christmas lights and ornaments to decorate mom's room for the holidays. We filled stockings for our mother and her roommate with Christmas candies and little tchotchkes—anything we could think of to brighten our mother's life. It felt woefully inadequate, but I felt satisfied that we'd done what we could.

What I didn't know was this would be the last time I would ever see my mother.

***

Back home in Texas, I welcomed my college-aged children and my brother home for Christmas. It felt so good to have my nest filled with the people I love so much. I did my best to enjoy the time with my family and avoid thinking about whether I had the big C or not. I reached into my bag of emotional tricks, and played the Grateful Game to help tame the whirlwind of thoughts that swirled through my mind. Some Al-Anon work and therapy helped with that, too. Letting go of what we can't control is so very hard! Especially when the stakes are high, like say, life and death. My mantra in those moments was, "If the outcome is the worst, I'll worry and stress then. If the outcome isn't the worst, I'll avoid wasting my precious time and energy."

On December 17, my husband came with me for my urologist appointment. After the exam, the doctor recommended an MRI and a cystoscopy—the initial procedure doctors perform to determine a diagnosis—which were scheduled for December 20 and December 27. It was hard not to be concerned about this.

On Christmas Eve, we received the MRI report, which showed no evidence of a tumor. My husband and I were so relieved! We believed this meant I didn't have cancer! I called my urologist's office and asked if they could cancel the cystoscopy, since the MRI didn't show anything. The nurse answered that the doctor wants to proceed with the procedure because MRIs don't always pick up everything and the cystoscopy would be more thorough. Well, that was a buzz kill! We naturally wanted to learn that we had nothing to worry about, especially during the holidays when my kids and my brother were home for Christmas.

Two days after Christmas, on the day before my 57th birthday, I had a cystoscopy that revealed a "lesion." I saw it on the screen next to me. It looked like a soft little flowy cauliflower. The urologist recommended surgery to remove it and send for a biopsy. That procedure is called a Trans Urethral Resection of Bladder Tumor, or TURBT, and they scheduled it for January 10. Because the urologist told us that many bladder lesions and tumors are not cancerous, we were still hopeful.

During this time between knowing and not knowing, I could and did enjoy many moments of wonderful, loving family and friend time. I'll give myself a B+ for that. Pretty damn good, considering. We enjoyed making our family's recipe for "Nuts and Bolts"—Chex Mix done our way. We enjoyed last-minute Christmas shopping, going to the movies, opening gifts, going for hikes with the dogs, celebrating two birthdays the week after Christmas, and generally having fun being together. When worry and fear crept in to my thoughts, I practiced some self-compassion (another skill I was working on) and acknowledged them. After that, I redirected myself to the present. Most of the time. Give myself a B/B- on that part.

My good friend Lori and I share the same birthday, December 28. We are both tall, blonde (well, at least originally, blonde. By 57, it required assistance to pull off my original color), and blue-eyed, so we referred to ourselves as "twins from a different mother." On our birthday that year, we met for coffee. We'd known each other for 22 years and celebrated our birthdays together whenever we could. That week of Christmas has never been an easy date to arrange, though; both our families have other December birthdays besides ours—just too much going on the week of Christmas! The joke was that we had one birthday cake that we would pass around to each person on their birthday. By New Year's Eve, everyone is just done with celebrating. Lori and I had fun hanging out together, talking and laughing. I shared my health update and wasn't too worried about it. I explained that my urologist found a "lesion" and sent it to pathology. Lori, a doctor, knew at that moment what I would later learn—a "lesion" is a nice word that doctors sometimes used for "tumor."

***

Meanwhile, work was extremely busy for me. The deadline for most insurance enrollments was December 31, so my calendar was full. We had some unhappy agents making negative comments on our company's internal social media page, so I felt some extra stress dealing with that and finding solutions. Our primary contact at EliteEdge had been quiet, which I hoped meant good news, but had low confidence that it was.

Extending an olive branch, I sent Christmas gifts to the EliteEdge Agent Health Care launch team, although our primary contact, Morgan, refused to respond or provide his address. As challenges continued with Clarity's systems through December, our corporate sponsor at EliteEdge was understandably disappointed and angry. Morgan went radio silent for weeks and did not respond to any of our messages. Because we had no idea what was going on with EliteEdge, I met with my Clarity colleagues, Dave and Jackson, the first week of January to map out a plan for how we would grow our business without the EliteEdge account. We discussed several ideas for how to find another company that employed thousands of 1099s we could partner with to provide health care. We figured it was over with EliteEdge.

***

On January 10, 2020, I had the TURBT procedure with Dr. Bee. All went smoothly, and he removed the "lesion." He was confident he had removed it all. He sent it to the pathology lab and scheduled the follow-up appointment for a week later. I went home with a catheter and bag and although I was a good sport, I hated it. Carrying a plastic bag around that has a tube connected to a catheter is not a glamorous look. Also, it's not comfortable. I wasn't happy.

Flashbacks from when I was six years old and hospitalized for bilateral reflux haunted me. I remembered all the times I had strange adults poking and prodding at my body in the most private area of all. In the 1960s and 1970s, medical professionals were not trained on how to talk with children to help them feel more comfortable, nor were parents welcomed into facilities to comfort their children. I recalled feeling like an inanimate object that doctors worked on, rather than a small, scared child. I remembered as if it were yesterday: the square, mint-green ceramic tiles on the walls, the slick terrazzo floors, the shiny silver and impossibly bright lights that hung over head, the sharp antiseptic smell of the hospital, and the seven or eight doctors at the foot of my uncomfortable examination table. I hated these memories and hated reliving them even more.

My follow-up appointment with Dr. Bee was on Friday, January 16, 2020. He got a pen and some notepaper out and started drawing a very basic picture of kidneys, ureters, and a bladder. As he drew, he described that I had Stage 1, high-grade bladder cancer. High-grade means aggressive.

Wait, *what?!* Was this is really happening? To *me?!*

Dr. Bee further explained that the cancer seemed most likely contained to just the inner lining of my bladder and had not made it through the wall or beyond. So that was good-ish. But this still meant I had an aggressive cancer diagnosis! He also asked if I smoked or worked around toxic chemicals. No, not unless you count toxic people. I count more than a few of those.

He recommended immunotherapy, which would occur every six weeks followed by another cystoscopy to check for cancer. Assuming none was found, this pattern would gradually stretch out for several years and then it would be just annual cystoscopies. One concern was that there was a worldwide shortage of the BCG immunotherapy I needed. Weird. What the hell?

I felt shocked and annoyed by the thought of the constant parade of yucky procedures for the next several years and beyond. It would be super uncomfortable and inconvenient, but not life threatening. And what was with the worldwide shortage of BCG?

Dr. Bee had a great reputation and was well-loved by the staff, so I felt confident I was in good hands. Even though the profile of a bladder cancer patient is a 77-year-old male smoker, I came to think of my diagnosis as "garden variety bladder cancer for a woman." As if I knew anything.

My health care plan, which also happened to be the one that we sell through Clarity to our customers at EliteEdge, included a second opinion from a board-certified specialist. Although I assumed I had garden-variety bladder cancer, I scheduled that visit. It didn't cost me anything. This was the first time I'd pursued a second opinion, but the service is free with my plan. Plus, it was also the first time I had a cancer diagnosis. Because I trusted that my urologist was experienced and knowledgeable, I assumed the second opinion was a formality and that the diagnosis and recommendation would be the same. I even felt slightly guilty for sending a signal to my doctor that I didn't trust him. (What the hell is that? It's my health! Just because my doctor wore a white coat doesn't mean I should automatically trust and not verify his findings!)

Dr. Bee enthusiastically supported getting a second opinion and commented that it's a common and smart practice for patients who get a new diagnosis, especially one as serious as aggressive bladder cancer. I arranged for the new doctor to access my medical records and scheduled a second opinion for January 20.

This was my first experience with a virtual doctor consultation, and it went better than I expected. The second urologist oncologist recommended another and higher-tech exploratory surgery to confirm if this cancer was in fact just Stage 1. He explained that 30 percent of Stage 1 diagnoses are really Stage 2 and that the treatment plans are completely different. The blue light cystoscopy, or BLC—different from the regular cystoscopy I initially had—that he recommended was pretty new and not available with very many doctors. I researched specialists who do the recommended procedure and found none near my hometown of Austin. That surprised me, since Austin had more than one million people and was a high-tech, highly educated city.

I kept investigating and found one doctor in San Antonio and two in Houston who did BLC. I wondered if I should schedule appointments with all of them or ask the second specialist which doctor he recommended— all new and unpleasant territory for me. I decided to send my medical records to each of them and see who responded first as my next step for booking an appointment. I also sent the names of the three specialists to the second doctor to see if he could recommend any of them. He responded that he could recommend the doctors at Baylor White and MD Anderson. I submitted my medical records to both hospitals and hoped at least one would respond.

On January 26, Dr. Bee's office called to let me know BCG immunotherapy was available and asked if I was ready to start treatment the next day. I felt a little bit pressured from the nurse because there was such a shortage of the drug. But I knew I needed to get more information rather than hurry to start treatment just because there was some medicine available. Who knew "fear of missing out" could factor into cancer treatment? I knew I needed to confirm the stage and type of cancer I had because the treatment regimens vary for all the different stages and types of cancer.

Just a few days later, appointments started showing up in my calendar at MD Anderson for March 2 and 3. It was still mid-January and March felt like a long way off. At least my work was a welcome distraction, even if it was going sideways.

***

I heard about one unhappy customer whose last name was Whitaker, and wondered if she was any relation to the EliteEdge co-founder John Whitaker? Her name was Paige, and I called her to address the issue she encountered with the Clarity plan, which was a lack of availability of participating doctors in Washington state. I used my best relationship building skills to find out that Paige is John's ex-wife and more importantly, cofounder and current member of the board of directors of EliteEdge. I worked to win over Paige and made a personal connection with her. I asked questions, listened, reflected what she said, and proposed an alternate solution—a plan on the exchange. I found a plan that worked well for her, even though this effort earned Clarity $0.

Paige was very happy, and I knew this created a stake in the ground for rebuilding the relationship with EliteEdge. Now, I had a key stakeholder's ear and knew what I said to Paige would be shared with John, Morgan, and other leaders at EliteEdge. Excellent! If Clarity could create an advocate in Paige, she would share positive experiences with John and that would help make Morgan look better to his boss, among other wins. Knowing this, I shared with her all the glowing reviews from happy EliteEdge agents and how Clarity solved all the problems we initially encountered at launch.

Also knowing the importance of having Morgan's ear, I left him a voicemail and several messages sharing the positive experience I'd had with Paige, updating him on Clarity's progress on addressing the problems, and giving him the list of glowing reviews from EliteEdge agents. When I noticed that one of the largest industry conferences was coming up at the end of January 2020 in New York City, I asked Morgan if he and others at EliteEdge would be attending. It was a Hail Mary—and it worked!

Morgan responded that he and other EliteEdge executives would be in New York at the same time as the conference, but not attending because they would be there for something else. He shared that EliteEdge had accepted an invitation by the NASDAQ exchange to ring the closing bell on the last Friday of January. After I responded with appropriate enthusiasm, I received a message back that shocked me: "Would you, Jackson, and Dave like to join us for the after-party at the NASDAQ exchange?"

I already knew the answer to that question—but checked with Jackson and Dave just in case—and responded yes, we'd love to celebrate with them at the NASDAQ exchange in Times Square. I texted Paige asking if she would also be there, and if so, could I meet her in person. She was going, so we made plans to meet at the event. My husband's parents also lived in Manhattan, so we arranged to squeeze in a quick visit with them, as well as see a show and visit the Museum of Modern Art. We even got tickets to see *Hamilton*!

The NASDAQ after-party was jubilant, with all the top executives and leaders congratulating real estate agents and employees for doing such a great job to grow this company. EliteEdge now had 25,000 real estate agents across the world and was growing fast! I located Paige and in getting to know her, found we had several things in common. It was so easy to talk with her. We were about the same age, had children about the same age, were divorced from our children's father, and had discovered that life is too short to live any other way than fully authentically. She was now a yoga instructor and happy with her life, happy that John had found a girlfriend who was better suited to his drive and ambition. In fact, she was good friends with her ex's new girlfriend and they had spent the whole day together seeing the sites of New York! I even shared with her my recent frightening cancer diagnosis. Paige was very encouraging and empathetic. I could have talked with her all evening.

This event was the ideal opportunity for me to nurture relationships with my point of contact, Morgan, and to meet and develop relationships with other executives. I was in my element. Relationship building is my superpower! Using my best skills, I authentically shared glowing compliments of Morgan's work to his boss, the founder and CEO, John Whitaker. Morgan and John both beamed. Dave and I beamed. John shared the stories he had heard of agents across the country who were saving thousands of dollars. We exchanged ideas about how to leverage the value of health care to grow their business. Other executives joined the conversation and I seized the opportunity to introduce myself and share more compliments, excitement, and ideas.

Dave and I were thrilled to celebrate with this elite group of leaders from our largest client. After weeks of radio silence from Morgan—and thinking our relationship with this client was over—that evening gave us both renewed hope that this relationship would continue to bear fruit. We left the party on cloud nine.

At a breakfast meeting with Morgan the next morning, we brainstormed ideas, made plans, and plotted out next steps. The opportunity that we thought was lost was back and better than we could have hoped for. Just three weeks earlier, Jackson, Dave, and I were making plans for how to grow our business without EliteEdge. What an incredible swing of the fortune pendulum. We were so excited about the growing partnership with EliteEdge. Dave saw my superpower in its full glory and told me how impressed he was. He showered me with respect, appreciation, and opportunity for the future we could build together. He laid out his vision for maximizing my skills: "Run free and wild with relationship development." This was exciting and officially a career high!

Hours later, the reality of my health care crisis returned front and center. While enjoying an artsy lunch with my husband at the charming MoMA café, I received a call back from Dr. Bee. I explained that I had received a second opinion from a urologist oncologist who recommended a BLC to confirm which stage of cancer I had because the treatments varied so drastically between Stage 1 and Stage 2.

As I explained this to Dr. Bee, I actually felt guilty. I was telling him I didn't trust him and his expertise enough to proceed with his prescribed treatment and I felt bad for that and did not want to hurt his feelings! I know I'm not alone in feeling this way about getting a second opinion because I've talked with other cancer patients who've shared similar experiences. We see a white coat and want to trust them completely.

We feel like we are distrusting when we "step out on them" by getting an opinion from another expert. The curse of being a pleaser! I was almost more concerned about not wanting to hurt my doctor's feelings than I was about making sure I got the right diagnosis for my health. *Almost.*

I pushed through my discomfort because I knew my health was too important to take a sideline to my pleaser trait. My determination to advocate for myself looked over at my pleaser trait, nodded in acknowledgement, and passed her by on the way to taking control of my health: "Thanks, but we've got this."

Dr. Bee told me he respected and encouraged second opinions and agreed that the BLC would be a great next step, but he did not yet have access to the equipment. He reiterated that he was 100 percent confident he had removed all the cancer and that he thought BLC would be the standard in the future. Well, that didn't help me right now, did it?

I thanked him and explained that I found a urologist oncologist at MD Anderson who could do the BLC and had scheduled it for March 3, 2020. That meant I would hold off on proceeding with BCG treatment until I heard what the oncologists at MD Anderson recommended. I told Dr. Bee that I understood that there was no way to know when BCG would be available again because of the worldwide shortage.

And just why was there a worldwide shortage of something so beneficial to cancer patients? The answer was because BCG was only manufactured by one company in the United States and it wasn't profitable enough to increase production. Score one for capitalism, zero for humanity.

As we left NYC for home, I felt as if I were teetering just on the right side of the emotional chasm I had been navigating between my health and my work. I was relieved now that I had the experience of "disappointing" my doctor out of the way. I felt great about advocating for myself. Work was on the upswing. Things were beginning to look up—as much as they could given my circumstances.

Chapter 4:
Worse News

From where I stood at the beginning of 2020, March 3 seemed like a really long way off. My next procedure was five weeks away, which seemed like a long time to wait to find out if my diagnosis was correct or if it was worse. "Aggressive cancer" ruminated in the back of my mind. I activated my "avoid worrying about the unknowns" strategy. If it didn't turn out to be the worst case scenario—more advanced cancer—I will have had saved myself a ton of needless worry and unnecessary cortisol production.

So, I chose to focus on the likelihood that the blue light cystoscopy would confirm Stage 1 bladder cancer and the plan would be to proceed with BCG treatment. I distracted myself by pursuing the exciting new opportunities for work and buried myself in those until March.

Because March 1 is my husband's birthday and March 2 is my daughter's birthday, we celebrated them both with a nice dinner out before we headed down to Houston's MD Anderson Cancer Center. Also on March 2, the CDC reported 124 cases of COVID-19 in the U.S.[1] We didn't think COVID was something to be concerned over at the time—hindsight is 20/20!

In Houston, we stayed with my ex's brother and sister-in-law, Steve and Paula, and enjoyed a home-cooked meal. Coleman and I got up early on March 3 and headed to MD Anderson. If you've never been, the hospital complex is massive and extremely challenging to navigate. It's like a confusing city with many different buildings and labyrinthine parking lots.

---

1 All COVID-19 statistics mentioned in this book are from the U.S. Centers for Disease Control and Prevention at https://covid.cdc.gov/covid-data-tracker/#trends_totalcases.

We found parking lot #7 and made our way to the Mays Genitourinary Cancer Center and checked in. It's a beautiful facility with many fish tanks, windows, and comfortable seating. Eventually, a nurse showed us to our waiting room and explained that a resident doctor would talk with us about prepping for the blue light cystoscopy, which was scheduled for the next morning.

The resident doctor was warm and friendly, so I felt a little more comfortable. She asked if I smoked or worked near chemicals. Well, no to both of those…again. I also explained that I had no family history of any cancer. After the resident spoke with us about the procedure, she answered questions and left the room. As I waited for Dr. Kamat, my urologist oncologist, to arrive, I practiced some deep breathing. I inhaled slowly and deeply, then exhaled slowly. *Inhale two, three, four. Exhale two, three, four.* I repeated this breathing and after what seemed like a hour, I thought about stopping, but I kept going, thinking that any minute now, Dr. Kamat would come in. Ten minutes went by, then 20. I stopped looking at my phone to see what time it was and kept on doing my mindful breathing. I felt like I'd been doing this forever. When would this doctor come in?

Finally, 40 minutes later, Dr. Kamat knocked on the door and entered the room. He was slim with a confident, but not cocky, air about him. He spoke with a balance of warmth and professionalism. He said he wasn't familiar with Dr. Bee and as he reviewed my records he concluded with a dismissive "Hrumph." That did not give me the warm and fuzzies. I mentioned that I couldn't find a doctor who performed BLC and was pleased to find Dr. Kamat could do it.

The next thing Dr. Kamat said changed my life forever: "We are not going to do a blue light cystoscopy. You have another form of cancer, and it is very aggressive, always recurs, and is always fatal."

Wait, what?! What was he saying?

My mind started spinning. I had to remind myself to breathe. I clutched Coleman's arm as I tried to comprehend what I was hearing. This was too big for me to process. I felt like I needed to hit the pause button on this really crappy movie that was my life. I wondered how I was going to find the strength to absorb this shocking news and make good decisions about the recommendations Dr. Kamat would give me.

He continued: "You do have high-grade urethral carcinoma. But you also have another very rare form of cancer that only occurs in 1 percent of bladder cancer cases, called plasmacytoid. It is very sinister and sneaky. Plasmacytoid cloaks itself to make the healthy cells believe it is regular bladder cells. It always comes back and is always fatal. BCG won't treat plasmacytoid, so we have to throw the kitchen sink at it. We have to do chemo, remove your bladder, and do any trials that are available. If we do everything, we have a good chance for healthy outcome. But we have to do everything."

Remove my bladder?! Chemo?! As in *lose-my-hair* chemo? No words adequately describe how I felt. Kicked in the gut, shocked, gobsmacked— not even close! I didn't smoke, exercised regularly, ate organic foods, and had even given up sodas. How could this be happening to me? I'd worked so hard to take care of my health! Cancer—let alone a rare form of bladder cancer—didn't run in my family. What the hell?!

I asked the same question as all cancer patients who don't want to undergo such an extreme treatment: "What happens if I don't do chemo and a radical cystectomy?" The answer was horrifying. "You'd have about 12–18 months to live," Dr. Kamat said.

I felt like I'd been kicked so hard that my breath was almost knocked out of me! My heart sank and I felt light-headed. In that moment, I felt myself shift inside. I partitioned off my overwhelming confusion and shock and set it aside so I could focus on listening to the doctor. I knew I needed to pay very close attention to what he was telling us, and I couldn't do that if I was freaking out, which is what every cell in my body that wasn't cancer wanted to do.

Dr. Kamat explained the plan and said that next, he would proceed with the TURBT, minus the fancy blue light to make sure all the cancer was removed. If that seemed to be the case, the next step was to schedule chemo. It would be three days in MD Anderson with several different "medicines"—chemotherapy—and I'd do this every other week for eight weeks. Then a 60-day break to recover from chemo, followed by a radical cystectomy to remove my bladder. And if there were any trials that I qualified for, I'd do those. Dear GOD!

"What are the replacement options?" I asked. Dr. Kamat explained, "The neo-bladder or a urostomy, where we take a section from your intestine and create a stoma, which is an opening in your abdomen that allows the urine to come out. We'll reattach the ureters to the stoma." This sounded like a terrible experience, obviously.

And the neobladder? I'd heard about this option and knew that it least was internal. He explained that the neobladder takes about a year to train and there is leaking for that time. Dr. Kamat wasn't recommending that. I asked him, "Well, can't we use like a pig bladder or a 3D printed one or *some* other option?"

He answered no and explained why. I don't recall exactly what he said because those weren't options so it didn't matter. Dr. Kamat reiterated that left untreated, the plasmacytoid would kill me in 12–18 months. Now I really didn't have any words. With a timeline like that, time to decide was not a luxury I had. With my handy emotional compartmentalization strategy in place, I took zero time to think about it.

"Do all the things," I told him.

Coleman has always been impressed by my strength and fortitude when faced with very hard things. He commented, "That's just like Margo to man up." To which Dr. Kamat replied, "Actually, I'd call it *womaning up*, because I see the women making the hard decisions to proceed with the chemo and cystectomy quicker than men."

The next steps after womaning up were to meet with another urologist oncologist, Dr. Siefkers. She explained the drugs that they would use for the chemo, and I still don't recall much of what she said. It felt like I was in an awful dream. She also asked if I smoked or had worked near chemicals. I asked her why the doctors kept asking me the same questions. She explained that it is very common for bladder cancer patients to have done

one or both of those things. Or worked with hair dye. I have had my hair highlighted off and on over the years. Could that really have caused cancer?

Dr. Siefkers answered our other questions and explained what to expect next. My convenient compartmentalizing of deep feelings of sadness and fear was only temporary. As Dr. Siefkers described the four different types of chemo they would use to kill the cancer, tears began rolling out of my eyes and down my face. Shock and disbelief were back to haunt me, and I found myself asking, "Why me? If I wasn't exposed to a lot of smoke, wasn't a smoker, or male or 77, and never worked in a chemical factory, why did I have cancer?"

"We don't know. Sometimes, it is just random," she said. "We've had patients who are vegan, run marathons, and live very healthy lives get bladder cancer, so it's hard to know why you got it, Margo."

This did not feel satisfying at all! Random? Not cool, cancer, not cool.

Dr. Siefkers handed me a big folder with many pages of information about the chemo treatments, the potential side effects, what to expect, and where to get answers. I did not want this folder. I did not want to need that folder. But I did, and as I looked through the pages without seeing them, my eyes welled up with tears again. This felt like a crushing blow to my entire world! The names of the four types of chemotherapy looked like they were made up by fifth graders: Dose-dense methotrexate, vinblastine, doxorubicin, and cisplatin (known as ddMVAC). I felt like she had given me a really scary and confusing textbook. The words looked foreign and I felt my whole brain glaze over in disbelief.

Then we left—shaken, shocked, and scared. We had originally planned to spend the night with Paula and Steve but shit just got real. All of my extroversion and golden retriever tendencies left the building. I sent a text to Paula and Steve with this new and terrible update. I explained how grateful we were for their support and hospitality but that we needed to have privacy to grieve and deal with this. Of course, they were extremely understanding and concerned for us as well. We made arrangements to go by their house to pick up our things and check into a hotel near MD

Anderson so we'd be close by to get me to the hospital for the TURBT procedure the next morning.

When we arrived at their house, they opened the doors and with tears in their eyes, and hugged us both. They were so caring and understanding. Paula gave me a bottle of holy water and told me that it works and to keep it with me. We felt very cared for but also like we needed to be alone.

After we got settled into the hotel, Coleman left to get some take out. We ate, and I won't lie, we hit the mini-bar too. *This all sucked.* Adding insult to injury, I had to stop eating and drinking by 10:00 pm.

As of March 4, 2020, 245 cases of COVID-19 were reported in the U.S. The news was filled with concerns that a true global pandemic was emerging. Which we now know was exactly what happened. Super cool timing.

Although we had to wait all morning and afternoon (with no food or drink) before I was called for surgery, the TURBT went well and Dr. Kamat said he didn't see signs of cancer. Phew! He was still considering this to be Stage 1, which was obviously good news, relatively speaking. We took the next steps on this new and frightening plan. We returned home to Austin, stunned and desperately trying to understand this new reality, blissfully unaware we were also on the cusp of the world's new reality, too.

PART 2:

Relentless Fights, Wins, and Losses

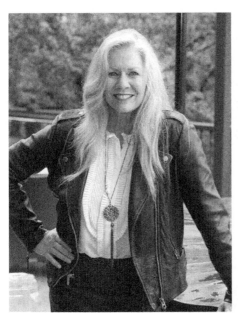

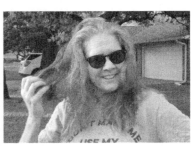

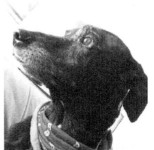

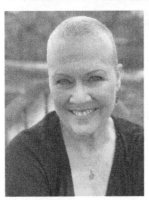

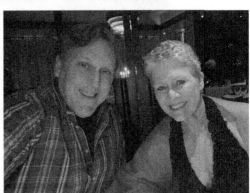

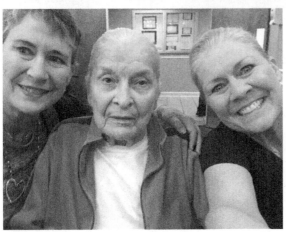

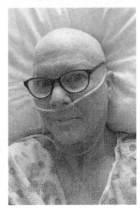

Chapter 5:
Buckle Up, Buttercup

Although this was not the worst news I'd had to tell my kids, it still hurt like hell to break this to them. I knew they would be worried for their mama. This is news you want to break face-to-face, if at all possible. My kids were both in college and my son was home for spring break that week. My daughter would fly in the following week.

Because my son was 21 years old, I gave him the news straightforward and was pretty thorough with the amount of information I thought he could handle. After all we had been through together, I knew my kids depended on me being alive and okay. I explained the new diagnosis and the treatment plan. I described the chemo plan, the surgery, and possible clinical trial. I left out the part about the 12–18 months that the doctors gave me if I didn't do all this treatment. Instead, I focused on that we caught this early, and it was still Stage 1, that the doctors were optimistic about the outcome. He took it in calmly, as was his new adult norm. I answered his questions and kept things real and somewhat light. He seemed okay.

Next, I called my 19-year-old daughter and took the same approach when I told her. I didn't want her to feel worried or afraid, especially when she was 1,000 miles from home. What none of us knew then was that after both kids returned home for break, they would not be leaving home for the next several weeks.

I texted my bosses the updated diagnosis and plan. Dave and Jackson were so very caring and supportive. They made me feel like my job was here for me, no matter how much time I needed to take for treatment and healing. I had been employed for just 10 months. I felt overwhelmed by and extremely grateful for the care and consideration I received from them. They were showing me the integrity I saw when I first interviewed with them a year before.

Meanwhile, the coronavirus was becoming a huge worldwide concern. On March 11, 2020, WHO declared COVID-19 a pandemic,[2] the first in more than 100 years since the Spanish Flu of 1919. On March 12, the news channels reported that Tom Hanks and his wife were diagnosed with COVID-19 in Australia.[3] The CDC reported 2,965 cases of COVID-19 that day.

***

On March 12, we drove back to MD Anderson in Houston. We met with the oncologists, and I went through several diagnostics to ensure I was healthy enough to withstand the extreme chemo treatment and surgery. And I was—my heart looked great, my vitals were all strong. I got the all-clear. The final step in preparing for the first round of chemo was to have a PICC line put in. That was a weird experience. The doctor came in and set up a sterile environment, which is very involved. Lots of sterilized equipment wrapped in plastic packaging. The doctor opened package after package and I thought, "This can't be good for the landfill."

She spread light blue surgery cloths all around me and set up her tools. She selected the large vein in my right arm—because it goes straight into my heart—and injected the needle directly into it. That did not feel awesome. It wasn't a tiny needle because it had to contain the PICC line itself. The doctor slowly fed the line up my vein and I could feel it! It was such a strange and unpleasant sensation. But thankfully it didn't take long. All that remained after she wadded up a mountain of blue papery stuff was a forked plastic tube with two different openings sticking out of my arm. One was purple and one was red. They dangled when I moved my arm.

Done for the day, we retreated to the hotel room nearby and watched some mindless Netflix show. I don't even remember what show we watched. Maybe the *Tiger King?*

---

2   https://pubmed.ncbi.nlm.nih.gov/32191675/.

3   https://www.cnn.com/2020/03/11/entertainment/tom-hanks-rita-wilson-coronavirus/index.html.

On March 13, President Trump declared a national emergency and banned travel from China, Iran, and Europe to the U.S. The CDC reported 3,916 cases of COVID-19 and 71 deaths in the U.S.[4] At the same time, my next step was a big one. We checked into the hospital for my first three-night chemo treatment. Because MD Anderson is a massive place with multiple giant buildings that together make up a small city, finding the right elevator in the right building on the right floor felt like a logistics puzzle. It was like checking into a hotel, but way less fun and far less luxurious. We settled into the room and the nurses took my vitals and hooked me up to the IV. We noticed that some of the nurses wore masks. We planned for Coleman to "sleep" in the "super-comfortable" fold-out chair in my room. The first bag of chemo showed up at 5:00 pm and they hung the pouch on the stand and connected it to my PICC line. The first night wasn't too bad. Coleman and I watched the news about this odd COVID-19 virus and wondered how it was going to play out. But the coronavirus was not our biggest concern.

By the next morning, I had a substantial headache and was feeling very tired. Coleman would put a cool washcloth on my forehead and that helped. A little. I felt miserable. When they brought in the final bag of chemo, the nurses were dressed in full hazmat gear. I'm not exaggerating. They were covered head to toe, and not because of this weirdo virus situation. That's how they were dressed to protect themselves from just touching the bag that had the doxorubicin, affectionately known as "The Red Devil." The medicine was so toxic, the nurses who handled it had to be protected from stem to stern. And that same medicine was going straight into my veins! I kept thinking that chemo seemed like barbaric treatment more fitting for medieval times. But this was the best treatment plan we had from the best bladder cancer doctors and saving my life was going to be worth all of this misery, right?

Having my husband with me during the four days and three nights at MD Anderson was so comforting. He would talk sweet to me, caress my hair

---

4 https://trumpwhitehouse.archives.gov/presidential-actions/proclamation-declaring-national-emergency-concerning-novel-coronavirus-disease-covid-19-outbreak/.

(while I still had some), change the cloth on my forehead, and love on me. Neither of us dreamed that this would be the last time he or anyone else would accompany me to the hospital for chemo or surgery for the rest of my treatments and for all of my follow-up scans and x-rays. Each day, more nurses and staff wore masks.

I watched from my hospital bed as the president delivered updates on COVID-19 in the U.S. I heard him talk about using virtual doctor visits as a safety precaution. As toxic chemicals slowly dripped into my body, I texted Jackson and Dave to tell them my idea for helping EliteEdge. We had a big opportunity to be proactive and innovative with our clients and offer our virtual primary care service, Teladoc, to their agents at a very low price. It would be a way to help EliteEdge agents immediately during this frightening pandemic.

***

By the time we checked out on Sunday, March 15, the first COVID-19 death in Texas was recorded[5] and MD Anderson established new COVID-19 precautions. All workers and patients were required to wear a mask. Patients had to wear masks to enter the building, have their temperature checked, and answer several questions about exposure to people with COVID-19 to get cleared to go to their appointments. Patients formed long lines to go through these new steps. Countless hospital workers were stationed everywhere to direct patients on exactly where to go and what to do next. The experience of staying at a cancer hospital for four days to get poisoned within an inch of my life to kill the cancer that was trying to kill me was surreal enough without a pandemic. I felt like I was in an alternate universe.

I slept on the way home and all day Sunday. That day, 9,656 cases of COVID-19 were reported in the U.S. and Las Vegas casinos and hotels began closing.[6] Each day after that, I felt a little bit better. Meanwhile, the virus was spreading fast, and COVID-19 cases and deaths continued to increase.

---

5 https://www.dshs.state.tx.us/news/releases/2020/20200317.aspx.

6 https://www.cnbc.com/2020/03/18/nevada-to-close-casinos-ban-dining-out-to-stem-coronavirus-spread.html.

My employers are outstanding guys and were incredibly supportive and understanding throughout my entire ordeal. Dave and Jackson sent a beautiful bouquet of flowers, checked on me, and offered encouragement and prayers. They also offered acceptance and flexibility. I felt so fortunate to work for compassionate and understanding employers.

The Monday after my first round of chemo, Dave called to ask me how I was feeling. After chatting a few minutes, he asked if I could estimate how much I'd be able to work each week. When I told him four hours a day, fewer at the beginning of the week and more toward week's end as I began to feel better, he was delighted!

Coleman noticed that when the phone rang with Dave's call, I was lying in bed. He observed that when I saw it was Dave calling, I quickly sat up and answered the phone energetically, "Hi Dave!" Coleman was impressed with how I could quickly go from out of it to up for my job. But after the 40-minute conversation with my boss, I collapsed back into bed and slept for hours. The first couple of days after chemo were the worst. I slept pretty much all day from the time I got home from MD Anderson until Tuesday. By then, I had started to feel a little better and was awake for longer periods.

Focusing on work was a wonderful distraction from the misery of chemo. It was just no fun to lie around and think about how bad I felt or worry about whether I was going to live or die. We know that a good way to fight the downward spiral of worry is to focus on something else. I've heard people say they feel better when they clean out a sock drawer. Doing some work that helped grow the company I work for was a rewarding escape from the reality of fighting cancer.

One of the few positives during all this was helping people solve a big problem in their lives. Our prospects and customers told us that health insurance had become one of the top stressors as self-employed people in the real estate industry. I worked for a company that provided a cost-saving solution. We were helping thousands of real estate agents save money and get better care. Making a difference in people's felt great!

I had scheduled a call between our team and EliteEdge's top executive Morgan for Monday, March 16, to pitch the telehealth concept. Because the call was the day after finishing my first round of chemo, I was exhausted and had chemo brain fog. As I pitched the value of telehealth for the agents, I felt my brain struggle to connect my thoughts. I was barely squeezing them out to form coherent sentences. My head felt so heavy that for part of the phone call I rested my head in my folded arms on the desk while Dave or Morgan talked. I felt *slow* and considerably less smart than before chemo. I didn't like how it felt at all. It was a very disorienting experience to notice that my brain was operating slower than normal, and so weird that no matter how hard I tried, I couldn't speed it up. Chemo brain is real and it sucks. After each round, my chemo brain improved over time, but never really lifted. And it took longer to recover after each treatment.

Thanks to Dave's normal brain operation and me occasionally spitting out something coherent, the call went well. Morgan loved the idea and agreed that offering telehealth at discounted rate to agents was worthy of a press release and marketing campaign.

As COVID-19 continued to rage, the U.S. saw grocery stores with shorter hours, reduced staffing, and toilet paper and hand sanitizer shortages. Social distancing was encouraged in public places, and numerous places cancelled large events, such as the City of Austin's signature music and film festival SXSW and Houston's rodeo. Things everywhere were shifting into unknown territory.

The uncertainty of what school would look like for my children loomed large. Their universities were each adding a week or more onto spring break while the school administrators scrambled to figure out a plan. Texas universities announced they would finish the school year online only and we began to hear rumors that classes for the rest of the year would be remote. My daughter, Rachel, a freshman at Colorado State, had flown home for spring break as my son, Read, a junior at University of South Carolina, entered his second week of spring break. None of us knew what the next months or rest of the academic year would look like for them.

Rachel is a creative gal, comfortable enough in her own skin to come home with blue hair. It looked really cool! She inspired me to dye my hair a wild color because it was going to fall out anyway. I decided to go big with bright pink! We had so much fun working the pink dye into my long blonde hair. It was some messy mama–daughter time that we enjoyed together. I was able to be present enough to enjoy this time with her and appreciate that she was old enough to share this moment with me. I didn't know what the future would bring or how much time either of us had on earth. But I knew that that moment was very good.

***

To avoid an extra three-hour trip to MD Anderson during my non-chemo weeks, I had blood drawn and my vitals checked at an oncologist near my home in Austin, who then communicated the results to my MD Anderson doctors. The goal was to determine if I was well enough to weather the chemo treatment. I always was. Turns out all of that working out and eating right made me stronger and more capable of handling the rigors of this aggressive regimen. Coleman and I wore masks to the Texas Oncology office in Austin—but we were the only ones doing so. We were surprised. If MD Anderson required everyone to wear masks, why wasn't Texas Oncology doing the same? One nurse even asked why we were wearing masks. I replied, "Because I'm a cancer patient and therefore am immunocompromised during a pandemic?!" I wanted to add, "Why aren't you?" My doctor heard we were wearing masks and did put one on to meet with us, so that was nice. Doctor's offices, hospitals, universities—pretty much everyone—were sorting out what their pandemic protocols were. It was ad hoc and inconsistent across the board. We were all doing the best we could.

By March 19, the U.S. had a total of 23,868 cases of COVID-19 and California issued a stay-at-home order mandating all residents to stay at home except to go to an essential job or shop for essential needs.[7] The order also instructed health care systems to prioritize services to those

7 https://www.gov.ca.gov/wp-content/uploads/2020/03/3.19.20-attested-EO-N-33-20-COVID-19-HEALTH-ORDER.pdf.

8 https://gov.texas.gov/news/post/governor-abbott-issues-executive-orders-to-mitigate-spread-of-covid-19-in-texas.

who are the sickest. Also on March 19, 2020, Texas closed bars, restaurants, and schools.[8]

Governor Greg Abbott issued an executive order that limited social gatherings to 10 people, prohibited eating and drinking in restaurants and bars but still allowed takeout, closed gyms, banned people from visiting nursing homes except for critical care, and temporarily closed schools. The executive order was effective through midnight April 3. On the same day, the Texas Supreme Court issued an order halting eviction proceedings statewide.[9]

By the following week I felt well enough to go for a short walk with my husband and dogs around the neighborhood. I had less energy than normal, but more than I would have at any time in the next five months. It felt great to get outdoors!

On March 23, Clarity issued its press release and our sales team began getting appointments for EliteEdge agents to enroll in telehealth. The pandemic continued to grow exponentially, with more than 62,087 cases in the U.S. and quarantining had spread throughout the country. No one could predict how this pandemic would impact business, real estate, or health care, but everyone agreed it would not be good. As a cancer patient receiving chemo treatment, I was immunocompromised and was especially vulnerable to the virus. Not cool, coronavirus.

On March 26, 14 days after my first round of chemo, I returned to MD Anderson for round two of chemo. The CDC reported the U.S. had 106,110 COVID-19. It was surreal how empty the highways were! With schools and businesses closed, quarantine was well under way. Only "essential" errands or trips were allowed. Cancer treatment counted as essential and there was about 5 percent of the normal volume of cars on the road. America was closed.

So were my hair follicles. I remembered the nurses told me that day 14 is when your hair starts falling out. That is so specific and accurate, and is exactly how it played out for me. I'd always wondered how that happens

---

9 https://www.texastribune.org/2020/03/19/coronavirus-updates-texas-economy-government-employees-
   telemedicine/.

with chemo patients. I learned that it starts with a little more than the usual amount of hair coming out when you brush—like 10 times as much.

I also noticed that my hair follicles hurt. Well, that's what it felt like. I don't know the physics of what causes that sensation. Did the chemo make the follicles weaken to the verge of follicle death, so they can't do their job of holding on to a strand of hair? It reminded me of when I was really sick and would go a few days without washing my hair. I'd have this same heavy hair feeling with the follicles hurting a little bit. So weird.

Because of the rapidly spreading coronavirus, quarantine and safety protocols were constantly evolving. Two weeks after my first round of chemo, MD Anderson no longer allowed any visitors, even for inpatient treatments, so Coleman dropped me off for three miserable days of chemo. I felt so empty and reluctant to walk back into the hospital for four days and three nights of misery all by myself. I *really* didn't want to be there nor did I wish to be all alone!

I thought of my kids and my husband. They are my "why," my bright shining North Stars in a sky of darkness. So, I took a deep breath and slowly opened the car door. I slipped the mask elastic behind my ears and picked up my heavy overnight bag. My husband asked me if I had my phone, chargers, computer, medications, toothbrush, etc., helping me make sure I had everything before I stepped into the hospital. Tears are running down my face as I write this. Even now, I can only write for about an hour at a time, because telling my story feels like reliving it and it was a terrifying, lonely, and miserable experience. However, *I am alive* to tell it because I kept going even when I didn't feel like I had the strength to take another breath or step! If sharing my story helps one other person keep fighting when they feel like giving up, then it's all worth it to me.

After kissing my husband through our masks, I got out of the car, closed the door, and turned to face my fate. I felt myself putting one foot in front of the other, willing my limbs to carry me knowingly to a really awful experience. I turned back and waved at Coleman and then cleaned my hands with hand sanitizer from one of the dispensers that were everywhere. Next, a greeter smiled at me. I think. It was hard to tell with the mask and plastic shield over her face, but it looked like her eyes were smiling and everyone at MD Anderson is super nice, so I assumed she was. She gave me a brand-new mask and told me to put it with the blue side facing out, then instructed me to get in the line, staying six feet from the next person. There were circle stickers on the floor showing people where to stand.

All of us cancer patients stood quietly, alone and six feet apart, waiting patiently for our turn to answer the COVID-19 questions through a strange plexiglass protective barrier. The worker asked for my ID number, and I gave it to her, along with my birthday and all the answers about not being exposed to anyone with COVID-19. The worker put the hospital bracelet on my wrist and then I got on the escalator. The Mays Clinic at MD Anderson has a very interesting and brightly colored two-story tree sculpture, and the escalator I rode took me right past it. It's cool looking. Not as cool looking as being at home *not* getting chemo, but you know, they try to make it as relaxing as possible and I appreciated that.

As I checked in for my blood work, I noticed that everything in the hospital was arranged differently from the last time I was there just two weeks before. The waiting rooms had about one quarter fewer chairs. There were more check-in stations and people making sure patients knew where to stand, where to go next. I noticed new signs everywhere with kind reminders about social distancing, washing hands, keeping the mask on—all the COVID-19 protocols. Some chairs had laminated signs that said, "This chair is unavailable." Everyone wore a mask and gloves; many wore plastic face shields as well. Another change that was annoying was that answering the same COVID-19 questions was required at every single checkpoint. But I understood why it was important. This was our new normal for who knows how long.

My right arm—the arm with my PICC line, which was the conduit for the chemo—started feeling strange near my elbow. I mentioned this to the technician who drew my blood, who recommended that a hematologist take a look. The nurse used a sharpie to draw an outline around the area on my skin that was red and warm to the touch. The doctor identified the cause was a clot and started me on a blood thinner medication. This was the start of an additional treatment that would involve painful shots directly into my stomach!

Afterward finishing my bloodwork, I found elevator R and made my way to the correct floor. I checked in and walked myself to my assigned room. I dropped my bag on the desk and made cheerful conversation with the nurses and techs. It's very strange to go into the hospital feeling good and come out feeling dreadful—knowing that this was on purpose.

The nice staff members got me settled and I waited for all four of my chemo chemicals to arrive at the same time to the pharmacy. Once that happened, they would start my treatment. Makes sense. Dose-dense methotrexate, vinblastine, doxorubicin, and cisplatin (known as ddMVAC) were my four. The four bags of life-saving poison finally arrived, and the nurses started me on the first one. As before, I felt pretty good through the first night and even into the next morning. My hair continued feeling "heavy" and my follicles continued to "hurt." Cutting my hair off was beginning to sound like it might be a bit of relief, but I still hated the idea.

I conducted our Friday sales meeting from my hospital room during my chemo treatment. And I was happy to do so. CBS News reported record numbers of unemployment benefit claims filed, the largest since 1982.[10] I still felt fairly decent, except for my slightly painful hair follicles. But that wasn't the case for long. By the next morning, I started to feel worse. I was tired, had a splitting headache, and didn't feel like eating. Especially hospital food. They try hard, but it really isn't very good. Add to that reduced "menu" options, due to COVID-19, and it was easy to pass on the meals that were delivered. Every hospital worker wore a mask, and many wore plastic face shields. I had to wear a mask, which added another level of discomfort, but I understood why. This was all just beyond lonely and miserable!

Chemo treatment round two went very similarly to the first one. During the first of the four chemo bags, I felt fine. Then as each chemo medicine was delivered into my body, I felt progressively worse. By the second night, I was feeling pretty lousy and longed for my husband's loving presence to

---

10 https://www.npr.org/2020/03/26/821580191/unemployment-claims-expected-to-shatter-records.

calm and sooth me. Talking and FaceTiming had to suffice, and they were poor substitutes.

After 25 hours of straight chemo, the nurses spent another 11 hydrating me with IV fluid. By that time, I felt terrible and looked puffy. God, I really hated this this! I wanted it to be over *now!* I tried to be optimistic and focus on being halfway done, but it was a poor attempt. I didn't feel hopeful. After checking out all by myself, I dragged my exhausted self out of the room, down the hall, and down the correct elevator so I could meet my husband at the "circle" drive where he would pick me up.

I felt like I couldn't take one more step. I wanted to just collapse where I was in the hallway. But if I did, that would create a scene and delay my arrival in the arms of my husband, so I told my feet to just keep moving. One step at a time. I watched myself slowly, so very slowly, moving closer to the glass doors at the end of the hallway. Freedom from this torture, reunion with my husband, and a three-hour long car nap awaited. Keep moving, I instructed my body.

Finally, I made it across the gauntlet! The familiar sight of my beloved in our black SUV waiting for me at the curb created a wave of relief that washed over my tired body and soul. I opened the door and gently eased into the passenger seat, collapsing in emotional and physical exhaustion. It felt *so* good to be back with Coleman, in our car, and heading back home. I fully reclined the seat, turned to face Coleman and said, "I hope you don't mind. I just want to sleep." As soon as I closed my eyes, I was no longer aware of the external world. I slept the whole way home.

Just like the first round of chemo, I felt exhausted and *struggled* to process a thought. Chemo brain is super annoying if you're trying to work or communicate. It was, a blessing if you just wanted to sleep or watch mindless TV. For some reason, the post-chemo mindless TV show I wanted to watch was *Criminal Minds*. First of all, it had interesting characters that I liked. It also had an easy-to-follow formula, although sometimes the real perp *was* the first unsub (unknown subject) presented. Typically, but not always though. It ran for like 372 seasons, so there were lots of episodes. I couldn't tell you what any of them were about.

***

Post-chemo exhaustion was more severe this time. My hair follicles were really bothering me, but I was too tired to do anything about it. My scalp still hurt, like when I've worn a ponytail all day. I planned to cut my hair as soon as I could sit up long enough to do it. My daughter helped me cut my hair and shave my head on Monday, March 30—the same day 188,731 cases of COVID-19 were reported in the U.S. We did a time-lapsed recording of it and it's still hard for me to watch. My daughter was sweet and loving and that made it a bit better, but I wasn't a fan of my GI Jane look.

***

The world was in such a strange place. The COVID-19 crisis presented a huge challenge. Businesses were struggling to adapt. No one knew what to expect and our largest client was no different. Morgan went dark again, as he and the other execs wrestled with the effects that the pandemic was having on their business. EliteEdge laid off hundreds of employees and we all anticipated a slowdown in real estate.

Clarity was already a virtual company before the pandemic and we all worked from home, so we were used to doing Zoom calls. EliteEdge had been virtual since 2009 and in 2018, purchased Vitality, a company that created online virtual environments for work collaboration. The leaders of EliteEdge were about to find out just how valuable that purchase was. The real estate company was uniquely set up to continue prospering during the pandemic while everyone else was navigating how to work from home and have Zoom meetings. Demand for virtual meetings skyrocketed and Vitality grew very fast.

After multiple failed attempts to schedule meetings with Morgan to keep the momentum going, I asked Morgan if Clarity could host educational webinars in the Agent Health Care Auditorium within Vitality, called "The Globe." He agreed.

At least Clarity could start the webinars, but there was so much more we could do to get access to the 25,000 agents and yet we had no support from Morgan and no access to other executives or leaders. If Clarity went around Morgan, it would infuriate him, and we would lose our key advocate. John Whitaker told the Clarity executives in the first meeting, "Stay close to Morgan, he's running point on this." For whatever his reasons were, Morgan was difficult at best to reach despite my best efforts. Clarity was blocked.

I didn't accept that the block was infinite and final. I spent countless hours researching the EliteEdge's websites (there are more than 20), scouring their press releases and news articles to find a "hook" I could use to re-engage them. I created a strategy based on what I learned was most important to them: Agent-centricity, transparency, agent retention, and growth by agent attraction. With no feedback from the EliteEdge team, I created a list of multiple activities to attempt to gain traction with their leaders. I knew I had nothing to lose, and Clarity had so much to gain; this could be so good for EliteEdge's business!

I tested many topics in the weekly educational webinars and invited EliteEdge agents through the virtual Globe WorkPlace, and email. I created the slide deck, scheduled, and managed the webinars, created the promotions for the weekly webinars, and tracked the impact throughout spring. I was hopeful the new marketing staff that would take over doing much of the tactical marketing work I was doing. I presented the first webinar on April 2—the U.S. had 270,891 cases of COVID-19—"How to keep COVID-19 from financially ruining you." With more than 50 participants and increased number of sales appointments scheduled with Clarity consultants, the concept was proven. Work wins felt good and took my mind off my battle with cancer. Thinking about solving business problems that help people was a welcome diversion. It felt good to see my efforts paying off.

***

It took an extra day or so after the second round of chemo for me to start to feel like a human. Add to that a daily shot in the abdomen that hurt like hell! Coleman would disinfect a tray, line it with clean towels and lay out the needle for the shot and syringes for flushing my PICC line openings. The flushing didn't hurt, it just felt weird to have what felt like a cold liquid push through my veins. My sweet husband had, up to then, been deathly afraid of shots and could never have a imagined he could gather his wits enough to give one to his wife. And give her those shots every day for months! He would psych himself up first. If I misread his state of readiness to administer the painful medicine, I would say, "Go ahead, I'm ready." Coleman would respond, "Wait! I'm not ready yet!" As instructed by the nurse via a FaceTime video call, he selected about a two-inch sized area of my belly flesh, gently pinched it together, stuck the needle in, and pushed the blood thinner into my abdomen. It *hurt!* We have a fair amount of nerve endings in our torso skin. Sometimes it hurt worse than others and left a bruise. But Coleman was a champ! When it didn't hurt as much, we'd joke that he needed to take a sharpie and draw a circle around that area for next time.

My brain fog remained, though. I continued to struggle to process, which felt as foreign to me as imagining myself as a math whiz. We all have different ways we are smart. The elementary and middle school my kids attended had a charming practice of identifying different ways kids are smart. My son was "body smart"—athletic—and my daughter was "nature smart"—she loved bugs and animals. Based on this spectrum, they sound like regular rocket scientists, don't they? Kidding aside, these were accurate assessments of my kids' interests, and somewhat predictive of their futures. My son played sports throughout high school and is pursuing a career in medicine and my daughter is studying animal sciences in college.

I had a pretty good feel for what my brain felt most comfortable handling. I was good at packing the SUV for road trips—"spatial smart." I could usually find my way around solving problems by connecting dots that weren't always evident to everyone. What is that? "Dot connecting smart"? Whatever you call that kind of smart, I no longer was. Listening to the description of a business problem, like when is the best time to send out a press release (not exactly a big ol' strategic mystery), I struggled to make the synapses connect to each other. I was using all my diminished mental power to squeeze a thought together. It was so frustrating because I couldn't keep up with myself. Honestly, my brain felt like a rusty machine attempting to crank after years of sitting idle in a dark, dank barn.

That may or may not make sense to other people who have experienced chemo brain, but that's how it felt to me. Because I was aware that I was struggling to underperform intellectually, I felt frustrated with my mental slowness. At one point, I remember thinking, "Is this what it's like to have a brain injury?" What's weird is that I also experienced an unexpected plus. My brain seemed to lack the focus, energy, and capacity to ruminate. Letting go was a whole lot easier! My brain wasn't capable of a whole lot of holding onto concepts of concern or deep thinking.

Um, good? But also, bad? Is my answer to inner peace an impaired brain? Surely, there's another way! I'm very aware that I am not a MENSA member or even sharpest tool in the drawer. However, I could hold my own in certain arenas, like figuring out timelines, and it was bizarre to struggle with that simple task. After each treatment, the brain fog began to burn off, little by little, I'd start to improve. But I never reached my original mental or physical capacity in between treatments.

Eventually I could take a slow walk around the block. That was the other thing. Most people would describe me as high-energy and I now felt more like the walking dead. This slow plodding was weird, but boy was I happy to get outside and see the blue sky, hear the birds singing, and join Coleman for a walk around the block with our dogs. This is another bonus I noticed. Enjoying the simple things in life is easy when you've been denied them for days or weeks on end.

Texas was in full lockdown by now, so getting out of the house was a big deal. I got excited if we had to go fill a prescription or pick up some groceries! Yay, an outing! Remember? It was surreal like an alternate universe in a poorly written sci-fi show with bad special effects. This was not *The Walking Dead*. This was more like, *Hoping to Go Outside Once a Week*.

Netflix and the other streaming services couldn't release new content fast enough. With billions of people stuck inside and starving for something to do, we lapped up every show the content creators made. And with a brain that is running on about 50 percent, I noticed I was more easily entertained. Another unexpected bonus to chemotherapy.

Because I was immunocompromised, we minimized outings to reduce exposing any of us to the dreaded virus. Remember, this was April 2020, with no vaccine in sight. It was full-on quarantine with 100 percent masks, social distancing, work from home, and don't go out unless absolutely necessary. Not exactly super fun times.

Also, with quarantine, supply chains were severely disrupted, so getting basics like toilet paper and hand sanitizer was a struggle. Tons of memes circulated about people hoarding toilet paper, sanitizer, and bread. It was ridiculous. My husband wisely decided that grocery delivery was a smart solution for us. Why risk anyone in the household coming in contact with COVID? The only problem was that the demand for grocery delivery was so high, the earliest delivery date was 10 days out. Well, that wasn't going to work. He geared up in the mask and gloves to go out into the scary world and bring back supplies, which we sanitized before unpacking.

I think it was funny that grocery delivery was booked solid for 10 days but alcohol delivery was available the same day. Explain *that* to me! We experimented with DoorDash, Grubhub, and several others.

***

I returned for round three of chemo on April 9. Each round of chemo left me weaker and for more days. I sported a buzz cut and had learned that a good way to remove as much of the hair as possible was to make packing tape donuts and rub them all over my head like a giant lint roller and it worked! I also learned why balding men wear caps. My head was always cold, so I wore a knit cap or a head covering. The satin leopard print pillowcases I ordered had arrived and I packed them in my overnight bag. The hospital staff thought they were fun and liked my "make the best of it and have some panache" attitude.

Another comfort item I brought to the hospital was a super-soft chenille blanket that a dear friend gave me. These little touches helped me feel connected to home and to the people I loved, which made being alone in the hospital slightly less miserable. It was still really awful. The nurses and assistants were all very nice and seemed to be even more accommodating than before. They knew we all didn't want to be there, knew we needed to be there, and wished we could have our spouses with us.

On April 9, 2020, the CDC reported 459,165 COVID-19 cases in the U.S. and 20,439 reported deaths related to COVID. The Department of Labor reported in the preceding week 6.6 million Americans filed initial claims for unemployment benefits. Nearly 17 million workers, 11 percent of the U.S. labor force, had filed for unemployment benefits in the last three weeks, as countless restaurants, hotels, factories, and offices had been forced to shut down to combat the spread of the coronavirus.[11]

The constricted supply chains and hoarding mentality of some consumers created odd shortages in toilet paper and hand sanitizer. A new social media platform emerged with short videos—TikTok replaced the void that Vine left years before. Initially, the young generations watched the endless supply of funny videos. Several talented people created funny TikToks about hoarding toilet paper, bottled water, and disinfectant. Some smart alcohol manufacturers began making hand sanitizer and selling it in one-gallon milk jugs. It smelled just awful—like rubbing alcohol but funky. My husband ordered a few different types and we all agreed it was nasty. We still have some left since we'd avoid that stuff if at all possible.

After my third round of chemo, I laid down in the car as my husband drove us home from the "shittiest spa in the world." I felt even worse than the last time. What the oncologist told me about feeling progressively worse after each round was true. Not sure how helpful it is to know that ahead of time, but I guess it might help for setting expectations with family and coworkers. I felt like absolute mush, mush, like an askeletal, barely-alive being. I'd compare myself to a tardigrade—a water bear—but those are oddly cute and I felt nothing close to cute.

They are, however, resilient. "Tardigrades are among the most resilient animals known, with individual species able to survive extreme conditions—such as exposure to extreme temperatures, extreme pressures (both high and low), air deprivation, radiation, dehydration, and starvation—that would quickly kill most other known forms of life."[12]

---

11 https://www.cdc.gov/coronavirus/2019-ncov/covid-data/previouscases.html for the total cases and deaths. Both cumulative charts on are that page. Unemployment data confirmed: https://www.cnn.com/2020/04/09/economy/unemployment-benefits-coronavirus/index.html.

12 https://en.wikipedia.org/wiki/Tardigrade.

Yeah, so maybe I am actually like those nearly microscopic creatures. I definitely survived many extremes during my chemo treatments, none of which had yet killed me. I think I'll give myself the new nickname, Margograde Thriversham, one of the most resilient people in the universe!

***

A twinkle of brightness during the dark storm of chemo came when Dave told me he was giving me the full bonus for the quarter! This allowed us to pay off our final credit card debt! We were recovering financially, even as we were purposefully dripping toxins into my veins with the goal of killing the cancer without killing me. I'll take that good and persevere through the hard.

Another win came in late spring when Morgan invited me to share the virtual stage with the new EliteEdge CEO, Jeremy Griffin, at the shareholder's meeting with three of their top executives. The event was a smash hit! More and more EliteEdge agents scheduled calls with the Clarity consultants and we saw double the monthly enrollments compared to the year before. I knew we needed to develop strong relationships with these advocates, so I sent thank you gifts to all three as a gesture of goodwill.

***

On April 24, I returned to MD Anderson for my final round of chemo. The CDC reported 923,268 cases of COVID-19 in the U.S. Standing on the sidewalk at the circle drive, I waved at my husband and walked into the ever-changing and unbelievably complicated COVID-19 precautions. I was glad that MD Anderson worked so hard to take care of immunocompromised patients like me. Getting treated for life-threatening cancer during a pandemic seemed like bad writing. I summoned my inner grit and checked in for my last round of chemo hell.

This one was the worst. I had grown weary of the physical toll, exhaustion, loneliness and pain. At least this was the last round and then I'd be done with chemo! I FaceTimed with my husband and kids, but I felt so weak and yucky that I didn't feel like even doing that—precisely why it would have been so much better to have my husband there with me. But *no!* Because of some stupid virus, my horrible experience with chemo and surgery was untenable. The headaches were even more horrendous and the hospital food even more unpleasant. Plus, the "menu" was now even more abbreviated because of freaking COVID. The sauteed spinach was actually just canned spinach served at slightly above room temperature.

The scale of my experience at the shittiest spa on earth ranged from heartwarming to sheer living hell. Every single worker at MD Anderson is trained so well to be empathetic, affirming, helpful, and caring. They understood how sad the patients were to be there for treatment without a loved one and they did their best to pour extra care onto us. As an extrovert and recovering pleaser, I found myself asking the techs, nurses, and doctors about their work and life. I'm naturally interested in getting to know people and finding out what they care about. I get a little jolt of happy hormones when I find a way to make someone's day a little brighter. They seemed to enjoy our interactions. Getting to know the teams of people who took care of me helped make the extremely difficult days and nights at MD Anderson a little less lonely.

By the end of my final round of chemo, it was the very end of April, and the whole country was in partial or total quarantine. I felt like a complete mess. The U.S. had crossed the threshold of more than a million cases of COVID-19. I was even more fatigued and so exhausted I could barely to walk. I had to use the tiny percentage of brain power I had left to tell myself to walk, reminding myself that the arms of my husband waited lovingly at the end of this walkway. My head felt like it was going to split open from the pain. My face was swollen and red, which is not a glamorous look for a bald 57-year-old woman. At least I didn't have mouth sores, because I followed the nurse's directions and swished the extreme saltwater mixture twice a day. Bleck!

But now I was finally finished with chemo! Slowly, I began to feel a little better, although putting up with the metallic taste in my mouth was harder after round four. Nothing tasted good! I had six weeks to recover from this harsh chemo regimen before I had the dreaded surgery. I was bald, bald, baldy bald! No hair meant my head was always cold, so I wore my trusty knit cap to bed—in the summer in Texas, because my head got cold in the air conditioning.

***

Thinking back on these four-day and three-night lonely and miserable chemo weekends, it seemed like a bizarre Dr. Suess story. (Unlike the evil Wickersham brothers in *Horton Hears a Who,* I may be a Wickersham, but I do not identify as evil.)

> *Corellton MaGoo drove his wife, Margul MaGoo*
> *to the MD Anderson Cancer Center Zoo.*
> *She was there to receive treatments*
> *they hoped would cure the scary sickness*
> *that in her poor little bladder grew.*
>
> *The world was consumed with the COVID*
> *Fevers, coughs, and headaches were no good.*
> *The virus was highly contagious*
> *spreading so fast and outrageous*
> *that inconvenient safety protocols they withstood.*
>
> *With sanitized hands and a mask on her face,*
> *Margul MaGoo walked into that big scary place*
> *donned the hospital gown*
> *got on the bed with a frown*
> *and accepted that days of chemo were her fate.*
>
> *The first bag of chemo wasn't so bad*
> *the second one left her feeling real sad*
> *the fourth was the worst*
> *made her head like to burst*
> *it was known as The Red Devil bag.*

The hospital food tasted like paste

her stomach turned over in haste

she knew she should eat

but the smell was no treat

so crackers for meals she embraced.

After eleven more hours of hydration

Margul MaGoo was feeling consternation

The hospital zoo

finished with MaGoo

and spit her out for her homeward migration.

Chapter 6:
The Dreaded Surgery

The week before my surgery, my husband dropped me at the door to the local oncologist office for my pre-surgery bloodwork. COVID-19 was in full swing, so a nurse in full protective gear greeted me in front of the elevators. She aimed a thermometer at my head, recorded my name and temperature, and asked me to sanitize my hands and replace my mask with a new one before taking the elevator up to the office. There, I stood in line, six feet from the next person. When it was my turn, I approached the woman behind the desk. There was now a huge piece of plexiglass mounted on the desk separating us. When she asked for my name, I enunciated as clearly as I could. It was hard to clearly communicate through that plexiglass while wearing a masks. Everyone was patient and tried hard to understand each other, but it was super annoying. Not as annoying as 36 hours of chemo, though!

I received the all-clear the next day: I was healthy enough to withstand the extremely complex abdominal surgery. Yay.

June 10 was my surgery day. It was a complicated surgery, requiring a team of doctors. Dr. Kamat was head of demolition: he and his team would remove my bladder, uterus, lymph nodes, and cervix, and check for cancer. Dr. Smith was head of renovation: he and his team would remove a piece of my intestine, repair that section, and create a new conduit that would direct urine out of my body through a permanent hole, called a stoma. Then they would connect my ureters to the new short section of intestine, and create the stoma. I would have plastic urostomy bags that would stick to my abdomen that would collect urine from the stoma. Those plastic bags have a little plug at the end and the way I would empty the pouch would be to stand up in front of the toilet, remove the little plug, and pee like a guy. More or less.

The doctors said there is not a more complicated surgery done to the abdomen and the entire procedure would take about eight hours. *Eight hours,* y'all! I would be in the hospital for six nights and seven days— by myself!

On this date, the U.S. had about 2 million cases of COVID. The country had 88 reported cases just three months before in March! That's roughly 24,000 times the cases in three months' time! At that point, we didn't know how this would play out. There was still no vaccine in sight.

Meanwhile, my mother was suffering with dementia and rapidly declining. It was hard to know how much since no one could visit her. The nursing home tried in complete vain to protect the residents from the coronavirus. They would move the COVID-19 patients to one area and try to keep them away from the uninfected patients. But of course, this was completely ineffective.

I mention this because it meant that my mom was not in the same room or bed for very long. They were constantly moving residents around. That added salt to the wound of denied access to visit and talk with my mom. Before I moved her into this nursing home, she was unable to operate her cell phone, so we turned it off. We relied on the land line phone in her room, which she shared with her roommate. Each of them had their own phone, but my mom either didn't hear it ring or couldn't figure out how to answer it, which meant we depended on the staff to facilitate a phone call. I'm sure I don't need to tell you that facilitating a phone call with a dementia patient during the COVID-19 pandemic was not a priority for those staff members.

But they tried. When we called to arrange to speak with our mom, we had to go through this song and dance or first ringing her phone. We knew she wouldn't pick up, but we had to start with this step. Then we asked a worker to check in on her and help her answer the phone. If she was awake. Dementia patients sleep a lot. Then there was the "Where in the

Nursing Home Is Our Mom" game, caused by reshuffling patients to "protect them from COVID." We made it happen every now and then, but that lack of contact left my siblings and I uninformed, frustrated, and worried!

Very rarely, one of the nice workers at the nursing home would use their own phones to set up a FaceTime call so Mom could see our faces and hear our voices. The stars aligned for a precious FaceTime call only one or two times between May and July. By then, I was completely bald, and explained it away by tossing out a carefree, "I felt like shaving all my hair off!" comment to her. She didn't seem startled, so I concluded she was continuing to decline.

***

The night before each trip to MD Anderson was always tense, and this night before my surgery was no different. I took a warm shower and let the water fall on my bald head and body for a long time. I looked down at my fairly smooth and flat abdomen. With some more discipline, I thought, I probably could have had a bikini body, but too late now. My bikini days were totally over. I allowed my brain to stop and focus on how my body was about to change dramatically, quickly, and forever. This is *not what I wanted!* In less than 24 hours, my body and life would be completely different. I did *not* want to have surgery. I did *not* want to have my bladder removed and have a plastic bag stuck to my belly for the rest of my life! I did *not* want to have to change the bag and deal with external urine issues—whatever that entailed. I did *not* want to be in the hospital alone, without my husband or children by my side. I did not want to be in the hospital dealing with God knows how much pain and discomfort. ***I did not want any of this!*** I felt angry that I had to make the choice between accepting all of this crap or death! Had I *not* had enough character development tragedies in my life already?! I don't think there are words to describe how desperately I wanted my reality to be different. Remove my organs or die. These were my choices?

I practiced deep breathing, visualizing positive outcomes, and relaxing. Sometimes, I had a little help relaxing with a stiff drink of grapefruit-flavored Deep Eddy to take the edge off.

The alarm is never a welcome sound, especially when it sounds at 3:30 a.m. for a radical cystectomy. But I was a realist and a grown up. So, I put my big girl pants on and packed for my trip to the shittiest spa on earth. The three-hour road trip to Houston was even less fun than usual, since I couldn't have any coffee, food, or even water. On the way home, I knew that I'd get to have all of those things but by then I wouldn't have a bladder. I guess you can't have everything all at one time.

The sun was just starting to rise over the horizon when we arrived at MD Anderson. Coleman pulled the car into the semi-circle drive and put the car in park while I put my mask on and gathered my things. Again. I kissed him through our masks and I took a deep breath. Exhaling, I very begrudgingly entered the hospital—accompanied only by a tornado of mixed emotions swirling in my head. I was scared, frustrated, angry, nervous, anxious. But also grateful I had access to some of the best cancer treatment in the world. A greeter checked my temperature and gave me a new mask. This rest of the standard operating procedures were in place, so I began the process of answering the COVID-19 questions, spitting out my patient ID number, birthdate, yada, yada, yada. No, I hadn't travelled outside the U.S. in the past two weeks. Coming to MD Anderson was the *only* place I went, besides my back yard. The world was in quarantine. No one was going anywhere.

I waited in pretty long line of patients waiting to be admitted for similar surgeries. We stood six feet apart. There were so many patients checking in for surgery! At least 20 on this floor at this time. All of us alone, with our one bag of things. The worker behind the plexiglass pleasantly asked for me for my patient number: 275-1784. I *knew* I'd never forget that number. (Months later, I'd totally forgotten that number. My brain wanted to forget this entire experience.)

The nice woman found my name on the list and said loudly, so that her voice could be heard through the mask and the plexiglass, "Room 13. Down the hall and to the left." Another masked worker handed me my hospital gown and socks. I imagined this was probably what it was like to get admitted into prison, as I numbly walked down the sterile hallway holding my just-issued garments. Once I found Room 13, a nurse nearby told me to change into the gown and socks and put my clothes into the bag on the desk.

Now this is one of those moments when I yearned for my sweet, loving husband to be with me and comfort me. He was so good at comforting me! I looked at my abdomen as I undressed and told myself, "This is the last time you'll look like this, Margo. When you wake up later today, you'll have a big red stoma on your belly with a plastic bag attached to collect urine. And that will be your reality for the rest of your life. *This is what it takes for you to have a rest of your life.*" I really, really, really *hated* having to have this life-saving, body-altering surgery! I really just wanted to get up and run screaming out of the hospital!

How did I keep myself from doing that? I reminded myself of my "why." My kids and my loving husband. And my family. And my friends. I couldn't wimp out and leave them grieving me. Especially my kids. They'd already lost their dad. I had to persevere for them. They deserved that. So, I dug deep and put on that stupid gown and those stupid socks and got on that stupid, uncomfortable bed. I called my husband and felt a bit comforted by talking with him. This was hard for him too! Many times throughout my treatment I thought about the impact my illness had on my family. This wasn't just about me. They were also worried, scared, and frustrated. My poor husband just had to just drop me off at the door at MD Anderson and drive three hours back to Austin, all the while trying not to worry about me. That's just not fair to do to a husband!

My "team" came in and everyone was very nice. They explained what was going to happen and as soon as the anesthesiologist started adding something to my IV to help me relax, I was out. Or at least I don't recall anything from that moment on. The next thing I was aware of is foggily waking in the recovery room, feeling *very* groggy. The super sweet nurse allowed me to use her phone to call Coleman and hear his voice. He was *so* relieved to hear the surgery had gone well and to hear me talking with him. I was still so sleepy. I asked the nurse if I could go back to sleep, and was a little surprised to hear her say, "Yes, of course." I thought they wanted to wake me up and I absolutely wanted to escape back to the land of deep slumber.

***

When I finally woke up, the nurses and techs were extremely helpful and caring. Most of the MD Anderson staff is like that! It's amazing that they can hire and train so many people so well. I was in a lot of pain and felt terrible. This was right after the opioid crisis exploded and now there was heightened level of sensitivity to prescribing any pain killers to people. Even those who have had their guts ripped out and rearranged! Not fair! The best they would give me was Tylenol. And all the Tylenol they could give me wasn't making a dent in the pain. I was so uncomfortable! I wanted my husband there to stroke my hair and fight for me to get me more drugs. But he was back in Austin, desperately wishing he could be with me to love on me and help me.

That we couldn't be together to comfort each other was excruciating. Being admitted to a hospital for a major procedure is stressful enough. Add to that the loneliness of having no one with you to comfort you or advocate for you. Add to that extreme pain and the sadness of permanent and unattractive changes to your body. It really did suck.

That first night after the surgery was extremely tough. If I had felt better and been more mobile, I might very well have bolted out of the hospital. All kinds of tubes were connected to various parts of my body. The new urostomy bag was stuck on my belly to the right of my navel. The bag was connected to the "nighttime bag" that holds a higher volume of urine. Taped down tightly to my right wrist was the IV dripping fluids into me continuously. Hey, at least it wasn't chemo poison anymore! To the left of my navel was another tube sticking directly out of my abdomen. This drained the fluid from the surgery site and into a little plastic container.

This whole setup grossed me out and made me feel so fragile, vulnerable, and sad. Did I mention that I was all alone? I felt so lonely. I wished I had some excellent pain killers like we could get back in the olden days. I especially enjoyed Vicodin and would have appreciated the distraction of feeling good that the drug would have provided. Tylenol was it, though. Whatever, universe.

***

I'll spare you some of the more unpleasant details but suffice it to say recovery from this surgery included many unwelcomed experiences. Nurses who focused on various specialties would explain to me what they were doing to me and why they were doing it. One came to show me how to care for my stoma and how to change the urostomy bag. I really did not enjoy that, because it made me look at my new body features that I didn't want to see. As the nurse laid out all the items I would need and explained the process that I would need to master and use for the rest of my life, I felt tears fill up my eyes and run down my cheeks. It just felt like too much! I felt so isolated with no one there to stroke my hair or reassure me. I was in pain, alone, permanently disfigured, and petrified. The nurses and techs were extremely kind and understanding, but they can't take the place of your own loved ones to comfort you.

I had my phone and my laptop to stay connected to my loved ones, but I didn't feel like sitting up or holding the phone. I felt wiped out and was content to just close my eyes and try to sleep. I say *try* because the constant parade of nurses and techs coming into my room to check my vitals, draw blood, replace IV bags, and empty fluid bags was almost comical. They pulled blood from me every two hours, so my hands, arms, wrists were covered in holes left by needles. It was nearly impossible to get more than an hour of sleep at a time! I focused on my breathing and eventually, in between blood draws, fell asleep.

The number of different doctors and nurses who came to care for me is more than I can count. At one point, one of my doctors told me there were a lot of people in the operating room to help with the procedures, which wasn't exactly comforting to me in that moment. I knew there were surgical teams in the operating room helping with my surgery and I fully understood that it was a good thing to have the best doctors and nurses available to care for me. But seriously, no one wants an audience for something like this. This was more truth I had to accept even if every fiber of me wanted to reject it.

MD Anderson is pretty freaking amazing at most things. Good TV viewing options wasn't one of them. A few movies were available, and I'd already watched them over the course of my four previous visits to this hospital. The range of channels available was not vast, but the range of languages available for watching those very few channels was oddly broad. You had the usual ones: Spanish, French, Chinese, and Japanese, but there were also Swedish, Vietnamese, German, Hindi, Korean, Arabic, Thai, and some others. Narrow choices, deep range of languages. It seemed like state TV to me.

The one other thing that I give MD Anderson fewer than five stars is the food. I get how hard it is to prepare thousands of meals a day around a vast array of limitations for cancer patients. On top of those challenges was freaking COVID-19. *Everything* during COVID was less than, including hospital food.

My taste buds were living on a different planet anyway, so I found nothing appetizing. I've never found it so easy to avoid food. I thought to myself, "having this strong of an aversion to food could really help me get to my ideal weight." Ridiculous! I know! I should have been thinking about how amazing it was that the fab staff at MD Anderson could and did save my life with some fancy treatment and surgery. Don't get me wrong, I *was* grateful for all of that. *And* I also wanted to be thin and attractive. I was raised during the "tall and skinny is beautiful" era. Christie Brinkley, Cheryl Tiegs, and Lynda Carter were the models to emulate when I was in high school, well before the "curvy is beautiful" era, brought to popularity by the Kardashians and Nicki Minaj. It's way better for society to view beauty as a wide range of characteristics and body types. But when the extra weight doesn't go to the areas that are prized for curviness, we are duped into finding it unwanted.

Adding insult to injury, this surgery had added bulk to the one specific area where I wanted to see less of me. Thanks, cancer. I marveled how the surgeon could remove multiple organs from my abdomen and yet my belly stuck out *more!* What the heck! Shouldn't it be concave now? Well, it wasn't. In fact, there was a whole new and completely unwelcome pooch below my belly button. I was so pissed! I'd worked so hard to keep a healthy and strong body, avoided having the mommy tuck, and now I had the opposite of what I wanted—an extra puffy belly *and* a big plastic bag stuck on the front of my abdomen. I was so unappreciative.

The workers would weigh me as part of the vital check, and I wondered why. Because I hardly could eat a bite, I did lose weight. Not gonna lie, I was pleased with the weight loss. They encouraged me to eat, but it was tough.

I had so much emotional baggage to unpack during my cancer battle and paired with a pandemic, a mother whose health was rapidly declining, and job stress and frustrations, I practically got whiplash from the range of emotions I had to process.

I struggle that sharing my grief about losing some of my attractiveness and youth seems shallow, but the permanence of these losses dawned on me during my treatment and recovery. I think this is something that all women struggle with as we grow older. I just had the added bonus of cancer and recouperation to contend with. As I recovered from emergency mode, I realized that some of the physical wreckage would be permanent, and that triggered additional waves of grief.

Women are conditioned to place a substantial amount of our individual value on how attractive we are. Losing whatever level of beauty we perceive we had is never easy. Looking at ourselves in the mirror and seeing an old person staring back at us is surreal. Men and women both struggle with accepting our aging selves as it is. When it's accelerated and exaggerated, it really sucks.

In talking with friends who have battled cancer of various kinds after age 50 or so, I hear a common refrain. The bald reflection is hard to accept and the change in our skin, the way it hangs on our faces, is even harder. Hair grows back for many of us, but our skin isn't going to reverse. I feel like I aged at least five years. Who the hell wants to fast forward the aging process like that? Or add some disfigurement? Yeah, great, I'm alive. And also, I'm very unhappy about some of my new reality. This was more opportunity for me to practice self-compassion. *This is hard and it does suck!* I worked hard to accept this. I also worked hard to find the positives—to find something to appreciate. At times, my search for gratitude found none.

I know that gratitude is a powerful healer. When I felt my lowest and least appreciative, I'd say out loud, as a way to remind and convince myself,

"I'm grateful to be alive, grateful for the love of my incredible husband, amazing kids, and wonderful friends. I'm grateful that my employers have been phenomenal throughout this journey. I appreciate that my husband and I are gainfully employed. I'm beyond grateful that this cancer took hold in my body and not one of my kids' bodies. I feel blessed to have had the ability and willingness to advocate for myself, to have a good health care plan that provided a lifesaving second opinion and access to the best cancer facility in the country. I'm grateful that Dr. Kamat accepted my case, that we caught it early, and that this extreme treatment regimen saved my life." Every word of that is true. And using this self-talk helped me generate that tiny slice of gratitude where there had been none—and it was enough! It's also true that I feel some anger, sadness, and grief about what I've lost. Truth and life can be messy and that's okay! We don't have to wait until life is nice and neat before we feel gratitude about the good things in it.

***

All those interruptions and the continual discomfort and loneliness made the time creep by so slowly. By the second day post-op, I seriously wanted a shower. However, I had all these attachments hooked up to me. So many tubes of fluids going in and coming out! It just seemed excessive. The plastic drainage container on the left side of my body was pinned to my hospital gown, the urostomy "night bag" hung on the right side of the bed, and the IV in my right hand was connected to a six-wheeled cart that reminded me of an all-terrain SUV (ATSUV). It even had a little basket, like on the front of a little girl's bike, that I kept my phone in. Any movement after this type of surgery and being attached to so many tubes is really difficult. Plus, I was in a lot of pain.

With help, I was able to sit up. To graduate from sitting up to moving me and my entourage of equipment was challenging. We made a plan for helping me get a shower that felt like preparing for an extended Arctic adventure in its complexity. A nurse helped me keep the hoses from tangling or getting caught in the wheels of my ATSUV. We moved the "night bag" from the bed to the basket of the ATSUV. Slowly—very slowly—and with the help of a nurse, I stood up. She helped me shuffle the five or six feet from my bed to the bathroom. Once in the bathroom, the nurse set out the towels and got me safely situated. She started the shower and explained how she would be right there if I needed any help.

It was the most pitiful excuse for a shower I can remember, but never have I been so grateful for one! After surgery and being in bed for a couple of days, I felt like a new woman! I mean, I didn't feel like the best *version* of a new woman, but it was all relative. The workers had changed the sheets on my bed, so I had fresh, clean sheets too! Opulent luxury, especially with my leopard print satin pillowcase and my soft chenille blanket that I brought with me.

Sleep came quite easily that night, although it was interrupted with the same frequency of intrusive interruptions. The staff were doing their best to take care of me and I did appreciate that. They were friendly, kind, and patient. I just kept thinking that technology needed to hurry up and progress so there was a better way to check the levels of whatever they were checking in my blood without sticking needles in me all the time. We can put a man on the moon, but we can't do bloodwork without needles? Elizabeth Holmes did have a great idea for creating a blood test that could provide mountains of data from just one finger prick, except for that pesky detail about the technology not actually being real. Still, it was a good idea.

***

How did I get though those miserable days and nights, all alone in the hospital room? At times, I felt desperate to leave and downright depressed that I was stuck there in this unpleasant condition. My will to live was nearly non-existent. I could understand now how very ill and elderly people say they are ready to go. That was new. Before all of this, I couldn't grasp how someone could feel ready to die. At certain moments, I felt ready to go. I felt as if I were only a faint ghost of the woman I had been before and felt barely alive. Anything to just make the suffering stop. During these moments, I tried to practice self-compassion and give myself permission to feel what I felt. This *did* suck! It *was* painful and I *was* lonely! It's okay that I hated this and desperately wanted to go home! It was normal that I wanted my husband with me. It was okay that I didn't feel like exerting any more effort to live!

My husband was completely accepting of whatever level of communication I felt up to. I missed him terribly and he wanted so badly to be there with me. Sometimes we texted. Sometimes we talked on the phone and sometimes we FaceTimed. Sometimes I didn't feel up for anything. But I always felt his love and support. *Always!* That was one of the keys to me getting through that week. And through the weeks and months before and after.

Feeling the love and support from my two children also gave me strength. They were 19 and 21 and mature beyond their years. We had been through *a lot* together and I was and still am so very proud of them! They are spectacular individuals. Authentic, caring, smart, and beautiful human beings. And they love their mama. They would check on me and tell me how much they loved me. I pined for them to visit me, but I comforted myself by focusing on that they were healthy and that I would see them in a few days.

I appreciated and respected that my kids took all COVID-19 precautions seriously during my illness. They were very good about wearing masks and socially distancing from their friends. My daughter would get together with her friends, but socially distance from each other, wearing masks. My son avoided leaving the house and played video games online with his friends instead. They each had friends who were less cautious, and it made them mad. They knew their mother was at a much greater risk. One of Read's friends made a trip to Daytona Beach with college friends, even though everyone advised against it. Daytona was one of the top Spring Break destinations for college kids and was known for having hundreds of thousands of students crammed together partying on the beach for a week. There was no social distancing happening there!

A bright spot in my days after the surgery was the festive bouquet of balloons that my friend Nanci had delivered to me the first day I was there. The balloons made me smile every time I looked at them. I felt loved and appreciated and was reminded how fortunate I was to have such wonderful friends. Nanci was part of my posse from the "old neighborhood," where I lived for my first 14 years in Austin. We'd raised our kids together, traveled together, and been there through thick and thin.

When I began to feel a pity party coming on, I would look at those balloons and remember how lucky I am to have such strong friendships. My heart filled with love and gratitude and that helped me get through the toughest and loneliest moments in that hospital room.

When I felt like I couldn't take one more second of this hospital experience, I made a conscious decision to focus on the relationships that made my life rich and warm. My husband, my children, my friends, and my family. "I am a wealthy woman," I would tell my children. I knew that I was also trying to convince myself. I wasn't as wealthy financially as I had been at other points in my life. I had lost so much over the past 10 years: our dream home on the water, my marriage to their father, and his tragic death when my kids were young. And now my hair and my bladder. *But not my life!*

Which still felt like a consolation prize. I mean, I have a *good* life. But I thought keeping my life was a forgone conclusion for at least another 15 or 20 years. I could never have imagined that my life needed saving at 57! I felt great and was healthy, so what the heck?

***

Finally, the doctors agreed to let me go home on day six, although they were strongly considering keeping me another day. I was so happy to call my husband and make plans for him to get me the hell out of there!

The nurses explained that they were making an exception to allow my husband Coleman to enter the hospital because he needed to be with me when the nurse gave me the final instructions on how to care for my new physique. I texted him as he was making his way to MD Anderson and when he said he was on the floor, I walked slowly to the hallway and when I saw him, I burst into tears. I've never been happier to see someone than I was to see Coleman in that moment. I threw my arms around his neck and buried my head into his chest and cried with relief and overwhelming emotion.

As the nurse showed us how to care for my stoma and surgical site, we took videos and photos. It just felt surreal, and I knew I wouldn't remember. *I just wanted to go home with my husband and get in my own bed.* It was

June 16, 2020, and there were more than 2.1 million cases of COVID-19 in the U.S. It was super annoying to wear a mask in the hospital for six days, by the way. Just one more unpleasant physical condition to endure.

Finally, we packed my things and Coleman took them to the parking garage so that all I carried with me were the balloons. The nurse helped me into a wheelchair and took me to the exit by the aquarium. She wheeled me outside where it was hot as hell, so we hung back in the shade, waiting for our SUV to appear. It seemed like we waited an hour, but I'm sure it was only a few minutes. There he was, finally! The nurse helped me get into the passenger seat, very gingerly. I thanked her for her help and waved, then she closed the door. *The relief!* I was in our car, with my husband, and going home! *Finally!*

I don't remember much about the drive home, except that as almost always, we stopped in Brenham for a bio break, the business term for a restroom break. When I walked into the house, the dogs greeted me with the enthusiasm of welcoming a soldier returning from war. To be fair, that's how they always greet us, no matter how long we've been gone.

My children hugged me tightly. I could tell they felt so happy to see me and relieved I made it through the surgery so well. I could not wait to luxuriate in the comfort of my own bed and new bed linens. I had ordered new linens so I'd have exactly this feeling when I came home from the hospital. I was very happy with that decision. The new sheets felt cool and smooth as I tucked myself under the covers and sighed a big sigh of relief. Home. Safe and sound, with my family, right where I belonged!

***

After I'd been home a few hours, Coleman told me about his experience dropping me at the hospital door and driving back to Austin, not knowing how I was doing in the surgery. He told me he paced around the house and wondered why it took so long and when the doctors would call. I can only imagine how hard it was for him to have had to wait so far away, knowing he wouldn't be able to see me for several more days. Coleman told me that when Dr. Kamat called to say I was doing great and the procedure was going well, he fell on the bed and cried. The amount of relief he felt was completely overwhelming! As my surgery continued, nurses continued to call Coleman to let him know everything was continuing to go well. The whole procedure took almost eight hours.

Coleman was the most attentive and loving caregiver I could have ever asked for. He made sure I took the correct doses of each medicine, which also included that lovely shot of blood thinner into my abdomen. You may recall that I had a new orifice in my abdominal region. My stoma was several inches to the right of my navel. That meant that I had a six-inch-wide sticker with a urostomy bag attached to it. This ruled out about a quarter of my abdominal real estate available for needle jabs. No fun for either of us. Besides taking care of me, Coleman was also working full time and taking care of the dogs. The kids helped with some of that as well. I felt grateful for them and them giving me the gift of not worrying if our home would run smoothly.

***

Being home with my family was amazing. I felt loved and cared for. I could finally sleep easily—no one was waking me up every two hours to check my vitals or stick a needle in my arm. No six-wheeled IV stand accompanying me anytime I needed to walk anywhere. No more loneliness, no more bad hospital food, no more uncomfortable hospital bed with scratchy, sharp-edged sheets. I relished this new comfort and luxury with the company of my family, all under the same roof. It was divine!

After I was home several days, I slowly acclimated to my new reality. My appetite slowly returned. What food did I want? Chick-Fil-A breakfast biscuits, the ultimate comfort food. My appetite still hadn't returned to normal, but it was getting better each day. My sweet friends had arranged meal deliveries, which was extremely helpful. Another friend arranged for us to have a housekeeper help clean and that was an amazing gift! I eventually felt good enough to sit outside and visit—socially distanced and wearing masks—with a few friends. It was better than no visits, which was exactly how many we'd had over the past few months.

About a week after my surgery, I felt okay to sit in a chair and make some calls for work. I continued trying to schedule meetings with Morgan and other stakeholders, like the marketing team, to no avail. I felt really frustrated and kept brainstorming for ways to get a response from a leader at this company.

I was trying to establish what my new normal looked like, including dealing with that freaking urostomy contraption. I have a hate/grateful attitude with it. At first, I needed Coleman to help me with all the steps required to replace the bag. It was a foreign world, with a lot of steps. And it wasn't—and still isn't—fun at all! I have sensitive skin and the large area that is constantly covered with adhesive complains constantly. It's very itchy under that giant sticker. It's amazing that entire industries provide supplies and support to ostomy patients. To this day, I hate changing the adhesive patch and bag. I've tried lots of different products to help my skin feel better, but how is it possible to for skin that is constantly covered by a large sticky patch ever going to feel normal?

Every time I tend to the urostomy, I remind myself I'm alive to complain about it. I'm grateful that the incredible team at MD Anderson saved my life with this extremely complicated procedure. I think about how grateful I am to have survived, knowing that so many people do not. Feeling grateful for the things I used to take for granted is an interesting experience. It's difficult to appreciate that which we have always had. I dislike the discomfort of the urostomy, yet I am grateful for the life it represents I have.

Chapter 7:
Highest Highs to Lowest Lows

I don't recommend having cancer during a pandemic. Cancer sucks any time! By the time my post-operation checkup rolled around on July 27, I felt anxious and worried that the CT scans would show the cancer had returned. It's such a weird sensation to feel physically fine and not know whether I still had cancer or not.

By the end of July, 4.6 million cases of COVID had been diagnosed in the U.S. and MD Anderson still wasn't allowing visitors to accompany patients into its facilities. My husband had to drop me at the door and then wait in a parking lot somewhere, because there were no places open where he could go.

I waited all by myself in the oncologist's office to find out if I still had cancer. I was tense with worry about what the doctor would say about my cancer status, after four rounds of intense chemo followed by radical surgery just six weeks ago. Had all of that worked? As I sat there trying to avoid freaking out and catastrophizing, I got a call from the hospital saying my mother was dying and I needed to arrange hospice immediately.

I reeled from this news. I felt the blood drain from my face and time slowed to a crawl. I reminded myself to breathe—*slow, deep breaths through my nose two-three-four, then exhale through my mouth two-three-four.* Repeat and keep repeating. This helped. Despite feeling slightly less anxious, I was aware that I also felt disassociated from myself, like a visitor in my body and this life. I looked at my hands, then my feet, and reminded myself that I am here, right now and breathing is a really good idea. Back to breathing. That helped me relax some more.

Finally, the oncologist came in. My anxiety spiked. Oh my God! What is he going to say? What is his body language saying? Is the part of his face that I can see behind the mask telling me anything about the news he was about to share? Does he look serious and maybe sad? I can't tell! With trembling hands, I called Coleman and put him on speaker so he could hear what the doctor was going to tell us. *Let it be good news,* **please!**

Dr. Kamat sat down and got right to the point. **No evidence of cancer!!** If you've ever experienced wondering if doctors removed all your cancer that is 100 percent fatal if not removed, you know what this feels like! The relief is indescribable! The depth of relief that I felt was beyond words. The intense and miserable regimen of chemo, followed by the most extreme abdominal surgery currently done on humans had *worked!* Thank God! That shit was *awful* to go through—and I had the fatigue and .25"-long hair to show for it.

In that very moment I was super-exuberant and grateful to be cancer free, yet only seconds before I had found out my mother has only days to live. I struggled with whether it was okay to feel happy about being cancer free or devastated that my mom was dying. Did I even have the capacity to feel both at the same time? I'd just had major abdominal surgery six weeks ago, for crying out loud!

My sweet husband picked me up from the circle drive and I got in the car and sank into my seat with total surrender. Drained from Mr. Toad's Wild Ride of life and death, I stared straight ahead. Should we celebrate my cancer victory, or should I call hospice and begin arranging for my mother's final days?

This was my "ah-ha" moment. I turned to Coleman and said, "We are going to take the next two hours to revel in the good news about my health. We are going to celebrate my health and our good fortune with some Chick-Fil-A and a milkshake, and talk about how relieved we feel as we drive home." It was so hard to let this amazing news sink in and believe it's true! I felt like we needed to give our minds and our nervous systems some time to absorb that this miracle has occurred!

We enjoyed those two hours of celebration. We talked about how relieved we felt. I felt like we had been triaging a massive multicar accident since March: more firetrucks, ambulances, and police cars than we could count, crunched cars everywhere, people in various states of injury bleeding and crying out in pain, medics racing to tend to the victims with life-threatening injuries. It was exhausting! We talked about how great it was to feel the weight of worry lifted from our shoulders. To feel the joy of me being cancer free! No more chemo. No more surgeries. No more shots in the stomach. It was a glorious two hours on I-10. I'm not aware if anyone has ever described driving on this notoriously congested interstate highway—the one connecting Jacksonville, Florida, to Los Angeles, California—as glorious, but I did because to me that day, it was.

At 12:15 pm on that hot July day in 2020, our two hours of feeling relieved and happy ended. I took a deep breath, exhaled, and dialed the Jacksonville hospice number. I marveled to myself, "How could this be my reality?" Well, it didn't matter, because it was, and I had no choice in the matter. I didn't want to make that call. But I couldn't let my mother languish at the hospital like she was. I hated that I couldn't talk with her. She had stopped being communicative in the past few days. When we FaceTimed, she would just look at the phone with what appeared to be empty brown eyes. But I don't think they were empty. I think she would have loved to have talked with me but couldn't because of the dreadful impact that dementia had had on her brain.

***

Watching mom's decline was especially hard because she was so smart! Sharp, quick-witted, and feisty, Susan McCutchin loved learning and loved going to school. So much so, that she kept earning degrees. She earned her Bachelor's in Science before marrying my father and as a social worker, putting him through law school. After raising kids and divorcing my father, she returned to school and earned her MBA with the goal of landing a better job. This was 1981 and she didn't get alimony, only child support for my young brother, who was still at home. My mother was a force. She was a woman who would have enjoyed life more if she'd been born a generation or two later.

Born in 1936 and raised in the deep south, success for her was defined as "marrying well" and raising a family. She was expected to go to college for two-years—also known as "finishing school"—with the primary goal of finding a good husband. That meant marrying a man who would make a good living and provide financially well for the family. Because she loved learning, she argued with her parents to stay in college and graduate, successfully convincing them to allow her to complete her degree. She earned a BS in Psychology from UNC Chapel Hill in 1958 and married my father, Ralph Wickersham, who attended Duke University, a couple of weeks later. They had met in high school in Pensacola, Florida. After they married, my parents lived in Durham, North Carolina, and my mother worked as social worker to support them while my dad attended law school.

Since I was a child, I enjoyed looking at pictures of my parents as a young married couple, living in Durham before I was born. They were such an attractive couple. My mother was 5'9" and very slender with long arms and legs and a small waist. She had dark brown hair, brown eyes, and olive skin, and would get a beautiful, deep tan in our summers at the beach. She had a beautiful face with high cheek bones and a gorgeous smile. My father was 6' 6" and played basketball in college at East Tennessee State before transferring to Duke to earn his law degree. He was athletic and striking with bright blue eyes and brown hair.

I thought they looked glamorous. Especially in their wedding photos. My mother wore a fabulous silk gown with long fitted sleeves and and a chapel length train. My father wore a white tux, black bow tie, and black slacks. As was tradition at the time, my mother's parents purchased a trousseau for her, which included very stylish outfits for her honeymoon and newlywed life. My parents changed into their "get away" outfits that made for very striking looking black-and-white photos. My mother wore a navy blue and white polka dotted dress, navy high heel stilettos, and a stunning wide brimmed navy hat with a white ribbon around the shallow crown. They looked like models and oozed with happiness and hope for a wonderful life ahead of them.

When I was a teenager, I learned about my mom's traumatic childhood. Her father was an alcoholic and would get mean with her and her brother, who was five years younger than she was. One wedding picture of my parents accidentally reveals the strain that my mother felt. Her father was so drunk at her wedding he could barely walk her down the aisle. The stunned and almost paralyzed look on her face says so much, as if she wanted to freeze that moment, wait for his drunkenness to pass, and resume the wedding once he was sober.

My mother was raised in a time and place where addiction wasn't acknowledged, much less discussed. Her mother did the best she could to keep her family stable, which meant keeping up the appearance of normalcy above all else. Although my mother well understood how painful being raised by an alcoholic was for children—and also how valuable therapy and mental health care were—she never attended Al-Anon meetings or truly dealt with life as an adult child of an alcoholic. It may be a common dichotomy—people who most need counseling go into the field of counseling.

My dad, Ralph Read Wickersham, carried his own pain from his father dying when my dad was just two years old in the late 1930s. His very smart mother, Margaret Read Wickersham, found herself a widow in the deep south, with two young children, during the Great Depression. She left her children with her aunt for two years while she attended Columbia University to earn her master's degree in teaching so she could provide for her family. There was no life insurance policy, no family money, and no government support available at all. She, like my maternal grandmother—Grandmommy, as we called her—did the best she could for her own family.

So both of my smart and attractive parents had a lot going for them and wanted to build a beautiful family together, but also brought a lot of childhood trauma into their marriage. My parents did the best they could. I did feel loved by them.

***

Fast-forward to 2020, the dementia that caused mom's decline would take her life. Even though her quality of life had suffered and even though I knew that her death was imminent, I still was not prepared for the devasting grief I felt. At this point in the pandemic, even a self-proclaimed optimist like me was struggling to stay positive.

As I spoke with the sweet hospice people in Jacksonville, Florida, I learned that managing the end of life compassionately during COVID-19 came with complications. There were different hospice options. My mother had been living in a nursing home. The managers and caregivers attempted to separate the COVID-19 patients from those who weren't infected, but in the end, all the patients got it. Including my mom. But this wasn't what was killing her. She was dying from advanced stage dementia, hastened by the pandemic. She had no fever, no symptoms, no cough, but she did test positive, so that triggered a very specific and complicated protocol for transferring her from the hospital to a location where hospice could care for her. She couldn't return to the nursing home to die because she was COVID-19 positive. She couldn't stay in the hospital, and she couldn't stay with me because I was half a country away.

Hospice had created a makeshift hospital facility for end-of-life COVID-19 patients. No one could visit her. None of us could physically be with our mom before she died. We could have flown to Jacksonville, but we would not have been allowed to visit a COVID-19 patient, even if she was our dying mother. We couldn't say goodbye to our mother. It was beyond heartbreaking.

I called my sister. We agreed our brother was not going to take this news very well. We placed a three-way call to tell him in the most compassionate way we could. We explained that mom had been admitted to St. Vincent's hospital with low vitals and minimal responsiveness. Once there, the doctors determined that she was dying from dementia and had only a few days to live. Because she was COVID-19 positive, they had to abide by a lot of limitations and protocols. We needed to arrange to bring her to a special hospice facility where she'd be cared for until she passed. Most devastatingly, we would not be able to visit her. At all.

All three of us struggled to accept what was happening, but my younger brother had the hardest time. As the oldest child with the fewest mental health issues, I was the point person and executor of our mom's end of life arrangements. So, mere hours after I'd learned I was cancer free, I was knee-deep in orchestrating the sad, lonely last few days of our mom's life. And we couldn't even see her. My sister even lived in Jacksonville, but absolutely no one was allowed in. Didn't matter if we were family and mom was dying. There was no way we could be with her! It was so very sad and tragic!

I made arrangements for her to be transferred to the special COVID-19 hospice location. Everyone says the nurses and caregivers who work with hospice are angels, and they are right. I don't know exactly how things were set up, but when I talked with a nurse, she explained that she would need to "suit up" so she could "go into" our mother's "room." It took a few minutes. I think it was a hazmat suit.

The nurses would take their phones and help us to "talk" with our mom. She couldn't talk or react, but we could talk to her. The hospice nurses say that hearing is the last sense to go, so they highly recommend talking, praying, and singing to the patients. How sad is all of this? So sad!

My sister and I called and talked to our mother with the help of the kind hospice nurses. We told her how much we loved her, respected her, appreciated her strength and determination, and valued the work ethic she taught us. She raised us to believe that our gender was not a reason for us to fail. We could do anything we set out to do if we did the work. She was a fierce mama bear to us, and we knew she loved us and did her very best for us.

Thankfully, we'd made mom's final arrangements three years before when we moved her to an assisted living facility. The minister from her church agreed to join us on a call with her, so we arranged through the nurse to do that. My mother loved music and especially enjoyed "Amazing Grace," so the three of us sang it to her. With tears running down our faces as we sang, we heard a very faint sound we thought came from mom. After we finished singing, we told mom again how much we loved her, appreciated her, and that it's okay for her to go when she was ready. By this point,

I was crying and feeling overwhelmed with sadness. The hospice nurse told us that our mother had made a sound like she was trying to sing! I struggled to stay out of the self-pity pit as I tried to communicate with my dying mother.

That was the last interaction I had with mom. She passed the next morning at 11:30, Monday, August 3, almost two weeks after her 84th birthday. The pandemic was still in full swing with no vaccines yet available, but we were no longer in lockdown and I was no longer immunocompromised, so flying to Florida was an option (although not one that was highly recommended). On that day, 890 Americans died from COVID-19 and my mother was counted as one of them, even though the virus wasn't what killed her.

Chapter 8:
Saying Goodbye to Mom

After the kind nurse called to tell me my mother had passed away, I sat on the edge of my bed and sobbed as my husband's strong arms wrapped around me. It was and still is so very sad. I knew and felt in my heart that I had done all that I could have for her when she died. That I never got to see her in person or say goodbye and that she didn't have any loved ones with her in her final days compounded my grief. Further destressing my siblings and I was that we couldn't have a traditional service for her and instead held a weird hybrid in-person/virtual service that didn't exactly go as planned.

It is still so hard to fully accept that our mother is gone. I still deeply grieve her loss and probably always will. I called my siblings with the sad news and we cried on the phone together. We talked about how we could do a service for her. There was no vaccine, but at least I was no longer immunocompromised.

My siblings and I wrestled with the decision of whether to have an in-person service or just a virtual service. I'd been doing video calls since before COVID-19 and it can work pretty well, but it falls hopelessly short of acceptable for important occasions like a funeral. My husband did not want me to risk traveling to one of the worst COVID-19 states but he lovingly supported my decision either way. I felt so comforted by his love and support.

My siblings and I were scattered across the country: I was in Texas, my sister was in Jacksonville, Florida, and our brother was in Roanoke, Virginia. The last time we saw our mom alive was in February 2020, before the pandemic was an acknowledged pandemic. The previous December when I flew to Jacksonville to move her into the nursing home, I had no idea it would be the last time I would ever see my mother. Her mind still had enough function and we had simple conversations, although she couldn't recall the name of the city where she had lived in for more than 50 years. It was an extremely sad and hard weekend.

We all felt strongly that we needed to be together to mourn the loss of our only living parent. We planned for a small, hybrid in-person/video service. I shared this plan with my sweet hubby and promised him I would take all of the COVID-19 safety protocols: wash my hands all the time, not touch my face, wear a mask all the time, stay six feet away from people, etc. He was completely supportive.

None of our over-65 relatives or friends could risk traveling and getting exposed to this horrible virus, which meant my mom's only sibling, her brother, Gene, couldn't come. None of the handful of friends my mom had could attend either for similar reasons. A few of our closest friends would attend in person and everyone else via streaming video. It would have been so much better to have Gene at the service, but this was before the vaccine and we understood he just couldn't take the risk despite him being a vibrant—but still 77-year-old—man.

This hit me particularly hard because Gene and I are close. He is the coolest uncle I could ask for. I have a small family, with one cousin in New York, and another cousin and my only uncle in Austin. Moving from Tampa to Austin in 1995 meant I had some family in my new town. Gene and his family were a big part of my life. We shared holidays together and they visited the hospital when I had my babies. I could talk candidly with Uncle Gene about challenges I had with my other family members, which was a great comfort—safe and warm. Also, I just really enjoy Gene's company. He's interesting and fun. I felt very fortunate to have him be such a big part of my life in Austin.

***

Staring out the window as I landed in Jacksonville, I felt disconnected from reality, as if I were in an awkward dream/nightmare state watching my life events unfolding in front of me. My mother was gone! I was here to attend her funeral with my siblings. I would never see her again. It seemed impossible to accept.

I hugged my brother so tightly when he picked me up at the airport. We clung to each other as if we were clinging to life itself. We were so torn up with grief. I knew this loss would be hardest for him. He was eight years younger than me and was 10 when our parents divorced. I was out the door to college, leaving him to essentially grow up as the only child of a working mother. My sister Karen and I had grown up with our parents together and our mom staying home with us. Craig had a radically different upbringing. Our dad wasn't present in our lives after the divorce, so mom was everything to Craig. He was very close with her.

As the oldest of the three, I always thought of Craig as kind of my child. I was so excited when he was born and couldn't wait to feed him, change him, bathe him, clothe him. Our sister was not as enthusiastic. She was only a year and a half younger than me. I remember once she was bickering with him and I fussed at her, "Why are you fighting with Craig? He's a five-year-old little kid?" Well, it turned out that she was suffering with undiagnosed bipolar disorder, which we didn't learn until many years later.

I feel protective of my baby brother, even though he is 6'6" and built like a linebacker. He's like a big teddy bear and seeing him so overcome with grief made me feel even sadder. It was more than we could take, and yet—there is no way to change what had happened. So we left the airport to grab some take out and meet at our sister's place.

That was hard for another reason. Karen struggled to live life and stay sober. She had extreme and rapidly cycling bipolar disorder, so life is very hard for her and we empathize with her. She had had hip surgery, so she wasn't getting around very well. Her place was a mess. Stuff was everywhere. Her cluttered studio apartment made it even more challenging for her mobility as well as for her to get organized. We saw her struggle to manage the basics in life, which added another layer of sadness to our grief.

The morning of the service, Craig and I picked up Karen. She needed a wheelchair, so we wrangled that thing into our mother's 17-year-old Subaru station wagon and drove to the funeral home. As we got out, I felt another wave of disconnection wash over me. It was so hard to act normally when we were walking into a funeral home for our mother's service. It felt like she should have been there with us.

One by one, our old friends wandered in and hugged us. Having them attend meant so much more to us than words can convey. These friends remember our mom when she was young and sharp and feisty. They were with us through many of our hardest times. Their presence as we tried desperately to come to grips with this overwhelming grief felt very loving and supportive.

The service itself? Clunky and awkward. How else can a Zoom funeral during a pandemic be? Hosting a hybrid celebration of life was so odd. We had technical difficulties, which is even harder to deal with when you're the grieving family members. The slideshow we'd made was tiny on the large screen at the front of this chapel. The microphone wouldn't work properly and we had a very difficult time figuring out where to place the laptop so the camera provided the best view of everything. The minister who presided was remote and that felt weird and disconnected. Through my tears and grief, I attempted to press the correct link on the same laptop for the piece of music we'd carefully chosen. I did not press the right links at the right time. Multiple times. So the music was played in the wrong order. It was not how we wanted this service to go. But we got through it.

With our brother in the middle, we sobbed and hugged each other throughout the service. It was a brutal experience on so many levels. Coming to grips with the harsh reality of our mother's death during a pandemic just weeks after I finished cancer treatment was all so overwhelming. What choice did I have? *I got through one freaking second at a time.* I just kept focusing on being present and feeling my feet on the ground and the warmth of my siblings' embraces as tears streamed down my face. All I could do was just let it happen, let this terrible tsunami of grief wash over me and not try to stop it or lessen it.

The in-person experience with my siblings and a handful of childhood friends felt immensely warm and therapeutic. We were so glad we had that time together to process the loss of our mother whom we had not seen in so many months. Craig, Karen, and I share our gratitude for our friends being there and supporting us. It meant so much that they'd come to support us during our mother's service.

***

We held a small reception after Mom's service, which in hindsight was a tremendous source of healing for my siblings and me. One of my friends reserved a beautiful restaurant across from the river for about a dozen of us to meet for lunch after the service. Craig, Karen, and I each had a couple of dear friends and their spouses join us. We sat at a big square table in a lovely room, surround by floor-to-ceiling glass that made the space feel both open and cozy. All of our friends shared stories about how awesome our mom was. They talked about how strong and smart and funny she was and how much she meant to them. That felt incredibly heartwarming.

Among the friends present was Craig's buddy Pete, his brother from another mother. They are both extremely intelligent, well-read, and very funny. As Craig's older sister, I can only describe it as adorable. Since I'm so much older than my brother, my friends had never met Craig's friends, so it was nice to see them all chatting and getting to know each other. What unfolded was almost magical. We laughed about old stories and antics and discovered some unexpected connections.

The coincidences were heartwarming. My friends Kathi and her husband Greg lived a few houses from where Pete's family had a beach house. They knew of each other's homes and families, but had never met. It was fun to hear them talking about people they all knew in common. Then my friend Anna asked Pete if he was any relation to Wade Hampton. "Yeah, he's my dad," Pete replied. "Oh my gosh! My mother was best friends with *your* mother!" Anna said. This launched another batch of funny stories, laughter, and much welcomed feel-good hormones for all of us. Anna and Pete talked about all the experiences *they* had in common.

As we reminisced about the good memories during this gathering of old friends and family, my soul filled and my healing began.

***

Long before dementia stole her vitality—when we were little—my mom could be fun and silly. Not perfect, by any stretch, but alive and vibrant. I remember once riding in the back seat of our station wagon after a trip to Publix. I saw her grab a Hershey bar and peel it open like a banana and eat it in a couple of minutes. She opened and ate another. I remember she ate four in a row, which was the only time I saw her do anything like that, as she always watched her weight, and cooked and ate healthy before it was trendy. No fried foods at our house. Sodas, cookies, and chips were occasional treats, which I later appreciated as an example to use for myself and to pass onto my own children. She was very active, athletic, and *always* slim—she played tennis and was an avid runner. But she did love her Hershey's chocolate and M&M's!

Another fond memory that comes to my mind is we always had kitties growing up and we loved them to pieces. One of our favorites was Samantha, who had a litter of kittens, including Pineapple, whom we kept. Pineapple loved buttercream frosting, so we had to make sure to cover unattended frosted cakes. But one time we forgot and we returned home to a cake that was as smooth as a block of ice. It had been licked absolutely clean! We knew Pineapple was the guilty culprit. I don't know how, but he survived the great buttercream frosting incident, and we learned the valuable lesson of covering cakes in the future.

My siblings and I could tell our mom stories to make her laugh, which was a lot of fun for us. One of our greatest hits was one story from one of our family's "Griswold" vacations. We'd load up the church-sized van with tents, duffle bags, groceries, and a cooler. The van was extra-long and had room for four rows of seats, but only had two. It seemed like an acre of space back there. We *always* camped everywhere we went, so we had a lot of gear to haul, aptly filling that giant space with tents, enough clothes for three weeks, a gas stove, and food.

The story starts with us driving through Death Valley in the giant van. Our extremely frugal father wasn't about to stop for food at a restaurant, so we made sandwiches while we drove. The person in the "way back"—the most coveted spot in the van—was closest to the cooler, and therefore was on the hook for making the sandwiches. It was July, we were driving 600 miles a day with minimal stops, and we were in Death Valley where it was 115 degrees. I was luxuriating in the "way back" by myself, so I was sandwich maker du jour. When I opened the cooler, I discovered the ice had melted. Everything that had been neatly packed into the ice was now floating. The ham, in a not-fully-sealed plastic container, was now soggy and floating in a sea of cooler water, along with the partially submerged, individually wrapped slices of American cheese. *Ewww!* Water had definitely come in contact with the cheese! The plastic condiment jars also bobbed in the tepid water. It was disgusting! But no way was my dad going to stop. As if there was anywhere to stop in Death Valley. It was squashy sandwiches or nothing for lunch that day, so I took orders for which waterlogged cold cuts my family members wanted. We didn't laugh about it at the time, but boy, did we make our mom laugh about it for years to come!

***

It's only natural to reflect on one's relationship with someone after they die. My mom left many impressions on me as I grew up—some are good, others are are painful lessons on how not to live and behave. I unpack those in a later chapter, but because this is my story of gratitude, I want to celebrate the valuable lessons I learned from my mom.

Build healthy relationships. With myself and with others. Relationship building is my superpower and has served me well in life and in business. My relationships have brought laughter during good times and comfort when it got dark. I entered adulthood with a handful of great, lifelong friends from high school, many of whom came to my mom's funeral. I had a wonderful relationship with my grandparents, who lived until just after I had my own children. The relationships we forge are the steel that supports us throughout life.

Celebrate. Celebrating the big and little moments in life was a big thing with my mom. Birthdays were usually fun and always included a white cake with buttercream frosting, especially if we kept Pineapple from getting to it first. Sometimes we made them ourselves and sometimes we got them from the bakery at Publix. My mother made sure that we always had "giftees" for birthdays, graduations, and Christmas. She made Christmas fun.

One of the most memorable gifts she gave me for my birthday was "Adopt a Manatee." The Save the Manatees organization offered this program to help raise awareness and money to protect this endangered species. Manatees are so docile and sweet. We'd seen them in the rivers and fell in love with their funny whiskered faces. "Success" was the name of the manatee that my mom "adopted" for me. She chose that manatee because she saw me as determined and successful at surviving a lot of adversity.

I must have passed this attribute down to my children because during my cancer battle, they helped me celebrate little moments. One afternoon, Rachel made a quick supply run and returned with a little surprise for me: a headband with silly, pink flamingo antennae! This may not seem like much, but it really lifted my spirits! She found them on clearance and bought them on a whim. It was this goofy little tradition we'd developed over the years. One year we wore Christmas tree headbands with multi-colored blinking lights. I sent a pair to my mother as well, so three generations of Wickersham ladies wore these silly things. The lucky person with a birthday gets to wear the brightly colored birthday-themed headband with 6" felt candles. My heart felt happy that my daughter had found a whimsical impulse buy that she knew would put a smile on my bald-headed face.

Get an education. My mother convinced my dad to let her go back to school to earn her MBA. That gives you some idea of the dynamic between them. She graduated with her master's degree as I graduated from high school. My mom later told me that she also wanted to go to law school, but my dad told her only one of them could and that he should because he was the man. She was so mad. It was also a long time ago, but still was a frustrating sign of the times she lived in.

I was so impressed with her for earning her master's degree. I marveled at her determination and discipline. She made an impressive countdown-to-graduation calendar for her final semester. It was on a large poster board and she mapped out all of her study time, project deadlines, and exams. She delighted in crossing each milestone off as she achieved them. I emulated her example when I went to college and have continued to use it throughout my life. When I had kids of my own, I taught them the same study habits.

My mom took me on a college tour that I still remember fondly. We visited Emory, Georgia Tech, and Furman in Georgia. She took me to visit Clemson in South Carolina and we toured Western Carolina in the mountains, Wake Forest, and UNC at Chapel Hill in North Carolina. We also visited Duke and University of Virginia in Charlottesville. I guess we didn't go north of the Mason Dixon line! When I walked onto the campus in Chapel Hill, I felt like I was home. The university had so much history, so many beautiful old buildings, so many interesting degree paths to explore and of course the gorgeous and luscious green "Quad," which teemed with students during changes of class and was a great place to hang out and throw a frisbee. Add to that, four beautiful seasons and this native Floridian was sold!

One really lovely asterisk to add to my chapter at UNC is that the same university president signed both my and my mother's diplomas. William C. Friday was president of UNC from 1957 until 1986. My mom graduated in 1958 and I graduated a semester early in 1984. Cool!

My mom eventually made her way into advising at the University of North Florida and earned another degree there, a master's in counseling. I liked to joke that she was showing me up, because I only have one degree. As recently as one year before she died, she still asked me to buy her non-fiction books, like *The Cloudspotter's Guide,* which explained the science, history, and culture of clouds.

Save for the future. My mother was fiercely independent and had a strong mind for saving and investing. She taught me how to save early on and through my teen years. That served me extremely well when I found myself responsible for 100 percent of my tuition and college experiences beginning my second year of college. She always encouraged me to pay myself first and start saving as soon as I could.

I earned $13,500 a year at my first job in 1984 and paid $300 in rent. I had no other income, so I was scraping by. Still, I started saving $50 a month and kept going throughout my life, which has provided financial buffer at a few different and challenging times.

Appreciate art. I loved that my mother took us to see the symphony. It was so much fun to get dressed up and go downtown to the Civic Auditorium and hear the Jacksonville Symphony play classical pieces I loved, and even those I didn't. I remember my mother always looking like a million bucks. She wore long dresses with elegant jewelry. It was such a special occasion!

An art museum experience that stands out in my mind as spectacular was a visit to the National Gallery of Art in Washington, DC. This trip was with just mom, Craig, and me. He was about eight and I was 16. Our dad was too busy working and he disliked cities and my sister was at music school for a summer program. The trip was pretty easy with the three of us.

We saw many works of art that I'd always read about and seen pictures of and there I was in the presence of these masterpieces. It was exhilarating! We were fortunate that Picasso's *Guernica* was visiting and on display that summer. That painting is enormous and incredibly moving! I think it's interesting that Picasso chose to use only black, white, and hues of gray. I also loved seeing Edward Hopper's *Haskell's House,* Andrew Wyeth's *Christina's World,* and other works by Degas, Gaugin, Manet, and Monet. Sharing our thoughts on the paintings as we looked at so many greats was a joy.

My mother noticed I was interested in drawing and painting as a young child and encouraged me to take an oil painting class, which I *adored!* I still have some of those early "works." I felt loved and encouraged that she supported my interests in art. She also gave me the opportunity to explore dance from the time I was four years old, and I discovered that I loved dance very deeply! My parents came to all of my recitals. Our treat after the performances, which ended very late, was eating pecan waffles at the ubiquitous Waffle House.

Travel. When the first National Lampoon's movie *Vacation* came out, I wondered if the writers had followed my family around because the similarities between Clark Griswold and my dad were uncanny. We would pack the van and go for long treks across country, seeing as many national parks as was humanly possible. *I loved it!* We started with a week in the Smoky Mountains when I was about six. Then we ventured farther and farther—Point Reyes on the California coast, Glacier National Park in Montana, and even Alberta, Canada. We saw Dinosaur National Monument, hiked in the Grand Tetons and Rocky Mountains, saw the tidal bore in St. Johns, New Brunswick, and the rugged Cape Breton in misty Nova Scotia, among so many other truly amazing destinations. I made a note to myself, "When I'm an adult, travel as much as I can!"

Pursue my dreams. My mother earned her MBA. She loved school and learning so much that she earned another master's degree and eventually became an advisor at the University of North Florida. I saw her fight for what she wanted and earn it. That's a powerful example to set for your children. She also encouraged my sister and me to have no gender-based limits on the boundaries for our dreams. I felt open to pursue what interested me and knew that my mother would accept and encourage me to achieve my goals.

We shared an interest in restoring old homes and purchased two dilapidated old houses in a historic neighborhood in my hometown of Jacksonville, Florida. We had so much fun working with the contractors to bring these properties back to their former state of beauty! My mom researched how to renovate historic properties and earned tax credits. She had the very smart idea of hiring a consultant to help us make the best decisions about renovation while still bringing the houses up to code. We successfully earned the 20 percent of the remodeling costs tax credit for each property and kept them for more than five years. We went for it!

***

As painful as it was to lose our mother, it was a blessing that she didn't linger in a state of utter confusion, unable to speak or react to us, like she was during those last days. I miss the way she was before dementia hijacked her brain. Like so many degenerative diseases, dementia is the slow goodbye that steals our loved ones from us one day at a time. Her quality of life had withered beyond recognition. I didn't want her to suffer. I felt peace about sharing my love and appreciation with her, and I was sure there wasn't anything else that could be done to save her.

Here's the thing. No matter how old or ill a loved one is when they die, we still have deep and painful grief to face. Losing my mother felt traumatic, like a knife sliced me deep in the gut. How can losing a parent, child, spouse, or loved one feel anything but traumatic? And just like so many others who have lost loved ones under similar circumstances, it still hurts.

It's a devastating feeling because loss is very real and final. It doesn't matter if they live to be 115, we are still going to miss them terribly and grieve that loss. When discussing the passing of an elderly relative or someone close them who was suffering, people will often say, "She lived a long life," or "It's a blessing that he's not suffering anymore." Those statements are true yet at the same time, offer survivors little comfort to their suffering and deep grief over their loss. Such statements are about the person who has passed. They are valid but unrelated to what the survivors feel. Grief is experienced by the loved ones left behind who are mourning the loss of someone very important to them, regardless of how much discomfort the person who died was in. Simply put, we miss them.

Accessing gratitude felt nearly impossible and I knew I had to find a way. When bad shit happens, I've learned to feel the pain, then I scrape the bottom of the barrel to find gratitude and I always do—regardless of how thin that slice of gratitude is, it's always enough to get me by. Sometimes that's all you need. I began writing down specific things I was grateful for. I'm grateful to the very special hospice nurses who wore hazmat suits to check on the patients who were dying. I appreciate that those angels allowed us to "speak" to our mom through their personal cell phones and sent us photos of her. I'm grateful for the dear friends of my youth who sat by my side at the funeral home. That my brother, sister, and I could share our grief in person together, imperfect as that was. That my husband and children were so comforting to me. That I took the time over the years to tell my mother what I appreciated about her. That I left no feelings unsaid. That I visited her every chance I could. That she and I worked together to publish her father's memoirs in the early 1990s, while both her parents were still alive. That we sent her a cake, ice cream, balloons, and silly hats for her 84th birthday, about two weeks before she died.

I did the best I could to be a loving daughter and to appreciate and enjoy what I could about our complicated relationship. I grieved the loss of the comfort she would have given me during my cancer battle if she could have. I wished she could have been less negative and less selfish about some things, and yet I was—and am—profoundly grateful I had her in my life for 57 years. I am a daughter who misses her mother. I wish I had more time.

Chapter 9:
Navigating School during a Pandemic

Little did we know that when we purchased our "empty nest" home in 2018—a small, one story, 1,647 square foot house—that it would become the mothership for our family during a pandemic, just a few short years later. We felt like smart 50-somethings, planning for our future as empty-nesters. Apparently, we were in fact trying to make God laugh, because what I just described is exactly the opposite of how we lived for two years during heights of the pandemic. It's how millions of families lived. It became our new normal.

We needed two separate offices for my husband and I to work and now we had two kids trying to figure out how to attend college classes remotely. And what they and every single other student of any grade learned was that fully remote learning sucked! Watching a professor teach classes to empty online classrooms through Zoom while all students were muted was less than ideal. As far as I could tell, all U.S. schools finished the 2020 school year that way and it seemed that 100 percent of students and teachers hated remote teaching and learning.

Like so many other parents, I worried that my college-aged kids would take a gap semester that would turn into never graduating. It was difficult to know how to counsel them. We all tired of hearing from every single news outlet, "These are unprecedented times." Yes, but so what? Our kids were growing up right now, trying to find a career path for themselves right now. It didn't matter whether we'd ever been in this situation because we were in it now and had to navigate it without a map. Everyone, everywhere was doing the best they could. It was so hard for so many!

My two kids were stressed and anxious about the disruption and uncertainty of their formative young adult years and looked to me for help in making decisions about what to do with these unfortunate circumstances. How was I supposed to offer them helpful advice when no one had any idea how to get through this?

Calling upon my experience with handling a few of life's curve balls, I relied upon my intuition. The details of the situation varied greatly from our previous challenges, but the same approaches would translate just fine. First and foremost, supporting what's in my kids' best interest was paramount. I knew from personal experience what it feels like when a parent puts their needs ahead of their child's—and I knew to avoid that. Maintaining and growing my relationship with my kids was also my top priority. If they chose a path that didn't feel good by my own personal mom standards, I would put our relationship ahead of my opinions. That's what protection looks like to me as they mature into young adults. Protecting our kids evolves as they grow. The picture of a momma bird sheltering her babies under her wing is the image that comes to mind when I think about protecting my children.

The overarching agreement in the U.S. was getting students and teachers back in the classroom for the fall. Throughout the summer, states brainstormed to find a way to open their doors, and universities debated acceptable solutions for the fall semester. Some kids decided to take 2020–2021 as the world's worst gap year. I totally understood that. The entire country was sick and tired of this pandemic. We all thought there would be a vaccine within months and then we could get back to "normal." *Ha!* Two years later, the U.S. was still struggling with redefining "normal." If I hadn't experienced the bizarre path that FDA-approved vaccinations took in U.S. culture and politics, I might not have believed it.

But in summer 2020, we all hoped we'd soon have a vaccine, and that life would regulate back to some semblance of normal, like the way it was before COVID. Oh, the summer of "us." We had no idea. It wasn't remotely anything like that. I'm still shaking my head at how naïve we were.

***

The week after my mother died, I was focused on work and helped my kids figure out their next steps for college. Read was on schedule to graduate in May 2021. The CDC and WHO were very concerned that students returning to campuses would create a spike in cases of the coronavirus. The University of South Carolina was considering a hybrid class delivery system: some online and some in person.

Without a vaccine, I wasn't comfortable with my kids going to back into the classroom. They weren't either. Read faced a tough decision. We spent a lot of time talking through his options. Return to Columbia and pay rent to attend most or all of his classes online or stay home and attend all his classes online and save $20,000+.

Neither of us wanted the dynamic or the outcome of him becoming that kid who never launches. My husband and I offered him a rent-free stay at home if he wanted to finish his remote classes from Austin and save the money he'd spend living in Columbia. I helped him weigh the options. He'd grown up so much in the past three years and it was an absolute delight to have him home. So, part of me wanted to enthusiastically plead for him to just stay here and finish his degree. And the mother part of me knew this needed to be his decision.

My son is not a partier and is rather introverted. He made a couple of friends, but really never found "his people" at South Carolina. One of those friends had already graduated and started a job, remote from Richmond, Virginia. Read felt like the social experience he would miss out on was not at all valuable, so he opted for the Finish-My-Undergrad-Finance-Degree-From-Home-Rent-Free plan.

One obstacle was that he'd signed a lease for an apartment, which started in August. We had some troubleshooting and problem solving to do. Because there was no clause in the lease addressing a pandemic that renders the need for housing useless, we started looking for people he could sublet his apartment to. Because I'm not a lawyer, I looked for friends who were attorneys who had knowledge of lease contracts. We needed some more resources. We reached out to our friend Michael, an attorney in Columbia, for advice.

He was ever-so-gracious and asked me to send him a copy of the lease to review. Turns out, he had some pretty deep experience in real estate law. Our other attorney friend was also helpful as we searched for ways to get Read out of this commitment.

Michael got back to us and essentially said, yeah, this lease is pretty standard and heavily favors the property owners. Our best bet was to find a sublet tenant to sign a sublet lease; then Read can get released from his contract.

We were concerned that demand for housing near campus would dwindle for the same reason he was looking to get out of his lease. I helped my son find groups on Facebook and elsewhere to promote the availability of the apartment. Eventually, he found a taker. Read had to discount the rent to get the new tenant to agree to sublet the apartment. In the end, he lost a few bucks and saved a ton, so that was a good financial decision.

***

Meanwhile my daughter was struggling with her own decision about returning to Fort Collins, where she, too, had signed a lease. She loved her roommate and had a great social life there. But like her brother, she was not keen to attend classes in-person before a vaccine was released and she wasn't keen to pay full CSU tuition for online classes. So, she decided to look for work and hope that classes returned to in-person for the spring semester. Everybody has to do what works for them. One kid decided to attend classes online from his room at home in Austin and the other kid decided to move back to her college town and not attend classes! As crazy as that sounds, I think they each made the right decision for themselves.

A couple of weeks before Rachel and I planned to drive her car to Colorado, she started feeling bad. Nausea, sore throat, fever. It sounded like COVID-19. She found a place and got tested on a Thursday. But it took at least three days for the results to come back. We quarantined her to her room and all wore masks in the house. That was super fun. We treated her symptoms with anti-nausea meds and kept her hydrated. But by late Saturday night, she was still feeling bad. She was 19 years old and had been listening to her 19-year-old friends who told her she needed to be seen by a doctor. And the only doctors available were at the emergency rooms at hospitals. Urgent care clinics had closed or had reduced hours. Everything was so much more inconvenient!

I felt very frustrated. My daughter was adamant about getting seen one way or the other—so I knew that I could take her or she would have a friend take her. I knew the outcome would likely be expensive and inconclusive, but she was an adult, technically. After talking the options over with my husband, I decided to take her to the hospital. And I was *not* happy about it because I knew it would be futile. Again, I focused on what was best for my relationship with my child. The $1,500 deductible we'd pay for this waste of time visit to the hospital was a price tag I was willing to pay to show her I was *with* her even when I didn't agree with her.

I'd had enough experience with hospitals and health care plans to know that they would give her a lot of tests, run up the bill, give her fluids, anti-nausea meds, and Tylenol and probably declare she had COVID-19. And so they did. It was more than $10,000 for four hours at the ER. EKGs, x-rays, pricey meds—the works! The result? They would not give her a COVID-19 test because she'd already taken one and was still waiting for the results and they thought she probably did have the coronavirus. Treatment for the virus was what we were already doing. So, thanks for basically nothing. That'll be $10K.

Her test results posted the next day and were negative for COVID! She had some other virus. Rachel has very dry humor and she told us, "At least I don't have enemy of the state virus." Gradually, she improved. We continued our plan for a fun mother-daughter road trip to Fort Collins, which I looked forward to and dreaded at the same time. It feels more permanent and grown up when they take their car halfway across the country to college, and much less like they are at an extended summer camp.

On the other hand, I love having time with my daughter and was excited about having hours and hours of time together in her car. I think most parents can relate to the mix of emotions we feel as we're packing our youngest child to move into their first adult apartment. Proud and hopeful for them and sad for our loss of them in our homes. For me, this was especially hard because I had just lost my mother three weeks before. I was only eight weeks post-op from my massive surgery and learning to deal with a whole new set of physical changes.

I was not ready to let her go. And there was no way I was going to stop her from going. I'd been on the receiving end of that parent child dynamic and it sucked. I wasn't doing that to either of my kids, even though I desperately wanted to stop them from leaving! A parent's love is a wonderful and sometimes painful thing.

Rachel's red Nissan Altima was packed and ready to set out at 7:00 am on August 19. It's a long drive to Fort Collins and we figured we'd allow ourselves two days to get there. We took turns driving and made regular stops to get snacks and take bio breaks. We laughed about how I'm always cracking the whip on family road trips to get everyone in and out of the pit stops fast. "That's where we lose the most time! Come on people, let's go!" We noticed that it was easier for the two of us to travel together than with the whole family. That makes sense; more people, more variables.

Rachel is always the DJ when we drive together, and we enjoyed a lot of great music together. We sang along together on the *Mamma Mia* songs and enjoyed a wide variety of tunes. If you've never driven through Texas, it's unimaginably big. We started from our home in Austin, which is in the center of the state, and drove for 11 hours before we made it across the state line into New Mexico. It's flat and boring in northwest Texas, which makes the road seem like it goes on forever.

With just another five or so hours to Fort Collins, we decided to push through and continue driving. We pulled up to Rachel's apartment building at about 1:30 am. I slept on an air mattress and Rachel slept on a pallet of blankets. The next morning, we shopped for the basics: a bed, basic supplies, and groceries. I enjoyed treating Rachel to a few items and we had dinner at a Mexican place. Rachel's bed couldn't be delivered right away, so we kept the same sleeping arrangements until I left. In the days that followed, I helped her get settled into her new life. One evening, we enjoyed an unusual pizza with cream cheese on it, and it was surprisingly yummy! We drank fancy coffees at one of the few coffee shops still open. We ran those last few errands before I had to leave.

***

As that time drew closer, I began feeling more and more sad. I felt like a visitor in Rachel's new life. Although she warmly welcomed me, this separation was another wedge between this mom and her daughter—which is how it's supposed to go. We raise our kids and if we do our jobs right, they become independent and leave to make their own lives. It also feels like a heartbreaking loss. Both exist at the same time, yet another of life's cruel dichotomies.

As I sat in the parked car, while my daughter and her roomie, Libby, made a Target run, I suddenly felt overwhelmed with sadness. The tears began streaming down my face and I couldn't stop them. I was overcome with feelings of loss as I saw Rachel settling into her first experience with life in an apartment at age 19. She was making plans with Libby for how they would cook together, entertain, care for their plants and fish. I had been watching her "adult" and saw that she was enjoying it. For that, I was pleased. I had done my best to teach her to live as a responsible adult and she was doing it right before my eyes.

I felt happy and sad at the same time, like I had when I found out I was cancer-free at the same moment I learned my mother was dying. And that had been only three weeks before! I felt overwhelmed, as if I couldn't handle this stew of diametrically opposing emotions.

And although I felt completely incapable of withstanding or managing my deep feelings of grief over the losses I'd sustained in the past few months, I remembered how awful it felt as a young college student when my own mother couldn't let me go and overstayed her welcome by spending two nights with me in my dorm room. Love for my daughter and my desire for her to have a happy and healthy experience as she left my nest was the best gift I could give her. I knew how much it would have meant to me if my own mother had provided such a loving release, there was no way I was going to let my own sadness stop me from giving her that gift no matter how much it hurt.

Isn't this the foundation of parenting? We do what we think is best for them, even when it doesn't feel good to us? I believe we parents work our butts off to help our kids have a good start in life to prepare them to launch successfully at some point. We're basically working ourselves out of a job from the minute our children are born.

When the girls returned from Target and saw that I had been crying (I tried really hard, but could not stop before they got back), I shared with them that I was okay. It's both wonderful and hard to see my daughter growing up. I didn't want them to worry and assured them I was all right. I was feeling the lyrics of the *Mamma Mia!* song, "Slipping Through My Fingers":[13]

> *The feeling that I'm losing her forever*
> *And without really entering her world*
> *I'm glad whenever I can share her laughter*
> *That funny little girl*
> *Slipping through my fingers all the time*
> *I try to capture every minute*
> *The feeling in it*

I had to let her go. And it's incredibly difficult. Rachel drove me to the airport and I hugged her then hugged her some more. And I turned and walked into the airport with tears running down my face. I didn't care who saw me or what they thought. Out of her view, I allowed the deep sadness of my youngest child moving into her own apartment and life far away wash over me. Deep down I was happy for her that she was happy in her new life. And I also missed her terribly in those same moments. That was a lonely and difficult flight home. I gave myself some self-compassion. *This is hard!* I told myself, "You remember how bad it felt when your own mother stayed too long, so you're not doing that. What a wonderful gift for your daughter, Margo!"

Then I remembered I had my oldest at home waiting for me and that helped cheer me up. Read and I enjoyed spending time together, talking about all kinds of interesting and sometimes deep topics. So, I focused on the bonus time I would have with my son, sponsored by the pandemic.

---

13 Lyrics by Björn Ulvaeus, Benny Andersson, performed by Meryl Streep and Amanda Seyfried, *Mamma Mia!* (The Movie Soundtrack Featuring the Songs of ABBA), CD, Polydor, 1774183, UK, 2008.

I remembered when Read left home pre-pandemic to drive to South Carolina for his junior year, I started crying as soon as the door closed. My daughter was still living at home and said, "Why are you crying now? You didn't when you first left him at school." She was right. The summer after Read's high school graduation was a little stressful. He was ready to go and was behaving in some obstreperous ways, which made me think it was time for him to go. In the two years since, he had matured quite a bit and was an absolute delight to be around and I already missed him. I replied, "Well, he's nice now," which provided us all with some comic relief. I chuckled at my own candor.

My gratitude for helping my kids navigate college during the pre-vaccine era of the pandemic flowed a little easier than some of my other chapters of challenge. I was grateful that the relationships with both my kids was so close and strong. I felt fortunate that they felt comfortable asking for my help and guidance. My heart was filled with appreciation for the extra time with my kids. I was glad we had the room (however compact it was) in our home to accommodate more time with them when they needed it.

Chapter 10:
The Hits Keep Coming

Rachel and I were having lunch with her friend Naomi and her mom in late May 2006. The girls were both five and had been friends since they were babies. Next to the restaurant was a Petco, which was hosting a dog adoption event. Naomi and Rachel saw the makeshift pens with all the dogs and begged to pet the puppies. Nanci and I told our daughters that we'd let them pet the doggies only if they behaved well at the restaurant. They were not especially well-behaved. But of course we let them pet the dogs because we moms secretly also wanted to hold the little fur babies.

I picked up a little black-lab-looking puppy and held her on my chest. She was so sweet and calm, not wiggly at all! I petted her velvety ears for a couple of minutes and gently put her back in the pen. When I turned to another pen to pick up another puppy, I felt a tug on my pantleg. I looked down and saw that adorable black puppy pulling on my pant leg through the side opening of the pen. Game over! She'd put a spell on me, and before I realized what I was doing, we were adopting this little dog into our family.

Nanci asked me, "Are you seriously considering this?" and I said, "Yes, I believe I am!" I called my then-husband and left a message for him: "If you don't want an adorable black lab puppy for Father's Day, you'll have to come down here to stop me from adopting her." He brought seven-year-old Read to meet us at Petco, and they fell in love with her as well! We were all defenseless against this puppy's charms. We named her Reagan.

She was such a fun puppy for the kids to have and became a fixture in our lives. One time, Read and I created an elaborate arena out of a building system for kids called Rokenbok. When we turned on the little vehicles to start playing, Reagan was instantly fascinated by the movement of the cars. She walked over to the setup and with one the swipe of one paw, destroyed the entire thing! Everything was in pieces. Read and I laughed and laughed!

She provided our family with one of our favorite activities: loving on Reagany. She slept on the bed with us, found a way to "steal" the covers, and barked at the wooden duck figurines on our coffee table. When Rachel would come home with a new stuffed animal, Reagan would simply take it from Rachel as if it were hers. She didn't destroy them, she just wanted them. We laughed at how she would bury Rachel's stuffed animals in the backyard. She once dug a deep hole and put a plush dolphin in headfirst, so just the fluke stuck out.

When we were moving from a rental house and had the van loaded to the brim, Reagan seemed concerned that we considered leaving her. She jumped into the van, somehow finding places to put her skinny feet among all the stuff. Normally, she would hesitate before jumping in the van, but that day she clearly had an agenda.

Our beloved dog had so much character, my kids said she seemed almost human. Reagan trained us to get her what she wanted. She had developed the habit of standing in the hallway, looking in at us in the family room, and barking at us. When she wanted treats, she wanted them *now!*

Another quirk that she'd always had was her obsession with shoes. She'd greet us at the door with a shoe—and sometimes a shoe and a sock, sometimes two shoes. When my kids were younger, we had shoe bins in the mud room where they were to deposit their shoes upon returning home. One week, I noticed there were more shoes around the house than in the bins. I asked the kids about it, and they vehemently denied skipping the bin. As I was cooking dinner one evening, I saw Reagan head into the mud room and my eyes followed her. I caught her red handed, gently picking out a shoe from the bin and trotting out of the mudroom with her prize! Laughing out loud, I called my kids and said, "I owe you an apology!" It had been Reagan the whole time.

Five minutes before I'd leave to get the kids from school, Reagan would start whining and go to the door. She knew it was time to get the kids and she wanted to ride with me to get them. That became our pattern.

Once we moved into a house with a pool, Reagan started a new tradition. She would chase the kids into the pool, pretend nipping at their heels! Peals of laughter and shrieks of delight told me this game was as fun for the kids and their friends as it was for our puppy dog. Our home was on top of a cliff and there were 120 stairs that led to a canoe dock on the creek. We had a couple of kayaks, so I'd take the kids kayaking up the very peaceful creek. It was like a park back in there! Reagany would come with us on an unsanctioned journey. She would swim and frolic in the water and then hop up onto some neighbor's property and run along the waterfront to keep up with us. If we came close to the mouth of the creek where it opened to Lake Austin, Reagan did something unexpected. She swam as fast as she could ahead of us and whined while swimming between us and the open lake. She did not want us going out onto the big dangerous lake! She was worried about us and trying to protect us, so of course we turned back. That seemed to make her feel less anxious.

Oh, and she was a runner! If she got the smallest window to escape and run, she would. And we couldn't catch her because she was so fast! It was beautiful to see her run. The greyhound in her made her look more like a cheetah than a dog when she ran. Once she escaped out the front door and ran with a herd of deer who had been running up the street. It was as if she had found her kin. She ran elegantly and fast, like they did and they were looking at her with bewilderment on their little deer faces, as if to say, "Who are you and why are you running with us?" Reagan was having a ball.

Another time when she got out (we had a real problem with her escaping), she found her neighboring and fellow truant dog buddy, Max. They were bad influences on each other and had a lot of unauthorized fun. Max's mom was a friend of mine and we would joke that our dogs were escaping to run away to the trail and smoke cigarettes together.

This puppy dog brought so much laughter and love to our family! By September 30, 2020, the U.S. had more than seven million cases of

COVID-19 and our nearly 15-year-old Reagan was declining. This beautiful creature was a member of our family and had seen us through some very difficult chapters. She was there through all the fun, celebrations, mishaps, difficulties, traumas, and challenges. When Coleman and I got married five years previously, Reagan was there. She adored him as much as I did. When my kids left for college, Reagan was still there, loving us, comforting me.

We made the difficult decision to gracefully ease Reagan across the rainbow bridge. I sobbed, my entire body and soul was so struck with this grief. You might think, "it's just a dog," but anyone who's ever had a pet companion knows they are just like part of your family and how difficult it is to say goodbye. I had only just buried my mother a few weeks before, and the pain of facing more grief and loss opened fresh wounds. During my life-threatening diagnosis and the months afterward battling cancer with all the horrendous treatments and side effects, Reagan had been by my side. She had been healthy and energetic until the last few weeks and then declined rapidly. I felt deep in my bones that she held on long enough to help me get through cancer and the death of my mother. Losing her hurt.

***

My husband's parents were living in New York City and enjoyed living on the Upper West Side in a senior living community. Well, they enjoyed it until the pandemic came to town, which it did faster and bigger in NYC. Like my mother, my in-laws were confined to their apartment. Masked workers, who had of course come from all areas on public transportation, brought residents their meals. The inevitable happened and a few residents contracted the dreaded coronavirus. Many did not recover.

We were very concerned for Coleman's elderly parents, but we were helpless half a country away. Just like there was nothing we could do about my mother. Coleman's sister lived nearby in Brooklyn, but could not visit them, either. Everyone with elderly parents worried about them getting COVID-19 and dying without being able to see them and comfort them. It was such a tough time for everyone. However, my mother and father-in-law made it through 2020 COVID-free, which was a blessing.

But in late October 2020, Coleman's father succombed to pancreatic cancer. When my husband told me the news, it didn't feel real. He had just enjoyed a lively chat on the phone with his father days before.

Coleman's father, CA, lead a remarkable life. Growing up in Taylor, Texas, he realized early in life that theater was his passion. His parents would drive him into Austin so he could see plays and musicals. They stayed in the car and waited for CA to come out after the performance. I love that his parents, who were from a small town in Texas and who never graduated from high school, were so supportive of their son's interests. This in the 1940s!

At age 16, he received a movie camera for his birthday. He wrote and directed a movie for his high school, called *Winner Takes All*. He cast the athletes and popular kids and knew how to get the most out of the actors. CA screened the movie for the principal, who instructed him to remove the kissing scene—such scandalous behavior was verboten for tender teenage audiences. CA agreed, but when the final movie was shown, the kissing scene somehow remained in! The audience loved it and the principal never took any disciplinary action.

CA joined the Army so he could attend college on the GI bill. The Army tested incoming recruits to discover their best talents and skills. After the tests, CA asked again when he would be directing plays to entertain the troops. The answer was after his training, of course. Upon completing the high-pressure training to learn how to use radar, CA asked when he begin directing plays for the troops and the response wasn't what he was hoping for. "Oh, we've spent too much money training you to land helicopters and you're really good at it. So, you will not be directing plays, Mr. Jennings."

The two relate: Directing plays takes competence, clarity, and confident decision making. So does landing a helicopter. Neither of those activities would benefit from an indecisive personality.

CA went on to earn his bachelor's and master's degrees from University of Texas at Austin. He began his career as adjunct professor of children's theatre at Blinn College. He knew that earning tenure required a lot more.

Professors needed to publish plays, earn PhDs, and win accolades. Ambitious and never shy of working hard, he moved the family to New York in the 1970s, so he could earn his PhD in children's theatre at NYU.

My husband has wonderful memories of living in New York. His family of four lived in a tiny one-bedroom apartment in Greenwich Village and Coleman had a window where he loved to hang out and play. He could see the Twin Towers of the World Trade Center from that window.

CA's hard work paid off and he eventually earned tenure. In 1980, Dr. Jennings was named chair of the drama department at the University of Texas in Austin. He was incredibly committed to his students and earned a reputation for being generous with his time and encouragement. He mentored scores of drama students and directed more than 50 plays for children. Relationship building was also CA's superpower!

CA loved his work and continued teaching until he was 83 years old. This is when I came onto the Jennings family scene and I could see his passion for drama and marveled at his energy. When I met them for the first time, Coleman's parents had just returned from a trip to New York. CA described the plays they saw, what he liked about them, what he thought could be improved. It was so interesting to me!

When CA retired, the drama department at UT hosted a two-day event honoring him and his career accomplishments. There were multiple activities, including panel discussions, short plays performed by students and faculty, and a keynote speaker. The impressive event included lunch the first day, breakfast the second day, and a very special closing dinner. Former students and colleagues shared stories about how CA impacted their lives and careers. One former student wrote and performed a song as she played her guitar. It was a very moving experience.

CA's health began to decline after he retired and by the time they returned to New York, in summer 2019, he needed a walker. His cognitive abilities began to slip and he slept more and more. During my work trip in January 2020, Coleman and I made sure to spend time with his parents. We enjoyed visiting them in their swanky new apartment. We had a very special family dinner in a private dining room in their building's restaurant. Coleman's sister, her husband, and children also joined us. It was a lovely evening. This would be the last time we would see Coleman's father alive.

Just weeks later, CA was diagnosed with pancreatic cancer. He decided to forgo the highly demanding chemo treatment that was recommended. By that time, he was very weak and frail and his body may not have been able to withstand the treatment. I knew from personal experience that it would have been a miserable experience for him. Coleman and I completely understood his decision. The doctors never said how long they thought he had and we all thought he had more than a few months. He didn't. We weren't ready to lose him. He died two weeks before his 87th birthday.

***

The parallels with my mother's death were unfortunately plentiful. The senior living community would not allow any visitors, so there was no way Coleman could visit his father before he died. Just as I had not realized in December 2019 that I was seeing my mother for the last time, Coleman did not realize in January 2020 that he was seeing his father for the last time. As his father declined, he desperately wanted to see his dad and hug him. It was impossible though.

Coleman had a really nice conversation with his father the Saturday before he passed. That was of some comfort to my husband, but nothing takes the place of visiting your parent in person before they complete their life on earth. And both of us, like so many across the world, were cruelly denied that basic gift before our parents died, just three months apart.

My heart felt heavy with grief, for my husband's loss and for mine, because I loved CA too. CA had been a wonderful, loving man who seemed truly happy to see his son happy in a new and healthy relationship with me. I heard him once say, "Thank God for Margo!" and it endeared him to me that much more. He expressed how much he loved his son and me, and he enjoyed seeing our marriage blossom. Coleman and I said early on in our relationship, "Coleman + Margo = So Much More."

CA's death was hardest on those closest to him—Coleman's mother, sister, and Coleman himself—as well as for everyone else who loved him. Everyone who lost a loved one during the pandemic knows how much harder it was to be forbidden from seeing them before they died. It was my turn to be there for my husband as he grieved the death of his father. It's so hard to see your spouse suffering with losses this painful.

Coleman's mother shared a lovely poem that a caring friend sent to her, that eloquently says it all:

> *We give them back to you dear Lord,*
> *who gave them to us,*
> *yet as You did not lose them in giving,*
> *so we have not lost them by their return,*
> *for what is Yours is ours always, if we are yours.*
> *And life is eternal, love is immortal,*
> *and death is only a horizon,*
> *and a horizon is nothing more than the limit*
> *of our sight.*

—William Penn

Chapter 11:
Doubling Down During the Storm

You've probably heard the mantra, "One day at a time." Some days, we have to take things one hour or even one minute at a time. Those are the tough days. And on those days, whatever gratitude we can muster is all it takes to help propel us through that moment. Just like processing grief or growing relationships, developing gratitude takes time. And what that looks like is different for each of us. Boy, it is so freeing to realize there's no one right way to grieve, process, learn, and grow. It's a personal thing and there's no wrong way to do it! Coming to this realization relieves the pressure to perform life in specific ways and also makes it easier for us to get through the tough times. You get through it by clutching onto whatever shred of gratitude you can find and it is enough to get you by. My attitudes and actions of choice—in addition to gratitude—are self-compassion, gratitude, grit, relentless persistence, and humor—and I clung to them all like a raft afloat in the ocean during a hurricane.

Cancer and the unexpected deaths of my mother, father-in-law, and beloved family dog during the pandemic were all so overwhelming they nearly knocked the gratitude right out of me! Work was an opportune distraction throughout this tumultuous time, and was a buoy for me to grasp onto. Any battle with cancer is emotionally and physically exhausting, and pile onto that a series of profound losses, and anyone can understandably teeter on the brink of despair. I was especially grateful to have a solid job with compassionate employers, which alleviated my worries about any financial burdens resulting from my illness. I was also grateful for the welcome wins that focusing on my work provided. I soaked up the gratification I received when real estate agents told us how much our health care plans improved their lives. Work gave me something else to think about besides cancer and sorrow, and instead gave me feelings of accomplishment and satisfaction. I liked how it felt to help people and achieve some success, even when I felt overwhelmed by fatigue and grief.

Early in the pandemic, and during my chemo treatments, I had worked to build on the successes that Clarity earned from the shareholder's meeting in April 2020. I had wanted to create video testimonials with the three EliteEdge agents who spoke at the meeting—at least they would respond to me!—but because Clarity's marketing team was committed to other projects, I got creative and did Zoom video interviews myself instead. I scheduled the interviews and hosted them with my bald head in plain view. I got some great video and quotes from happy agents, which was a solid win. It gave us something to talk about and work with.

EliteEdge, my largest account, had prepared for real estate to pull back and began laying off some of their employees. But the residential real estate market did not pull back, slow down, or even maintain a steady pace. Instead, it took off like a rocket! Demand for homes went through the roof. Everyone was shocked at how much demand spiked during the pandemic. Low interest rates and nowhere to go was making people want more from their homes. Working from home, home schooling, and stay-at-home orders required more space.

Parents who had, until quarantine, worked in offices were now all working from home and essentially homeschooling their kids—two things most parents didn't do before COVID. When Coleman and I walked around the neighborhood, we'd see people working from their RVs in the driveway. We'd see people exercising in their driveways because they couldn't go to the gym and very likely they were maxing out the square footage of their homes to accommodate working and learning from home. We'd see people add electricity to the sheds in their back yards. Moms and dads would be on Zoom calls from their kitchens or wherever they could find a decent place to work and kids, pets, and delivery people would interrupt regularly. We all got used to that, because we were all in the same exact boat.

All of the above meant that EliteEdge was growing exponentially, which was *very* good for our business. The fast growth phase of business is very fun.

This is especially true when your employer and your largest account have cultures of high integrity and collaboration. My employers were incredibly supportive and caring. Around this time, I had begun writing in my journal again and enjoyed thinking about gratitude. I had many things to appreciate: my family, friends, MD Anderson, my employer, my health care plan, a comfortable home, positive outcomes for the treatment and surgery so far, and a good job with a lot of opportunity to help people. Those teeny slices of gratitude were piling up. You can see why I wanted to get back to work.

Nine days post-op in July 2020, I sat in a chair and answered a few emails from my laptop. It felt *great* to be productive! Each day, I felt a bit stronger, so I worked a bit longer. After a year of intense work to build relationships with EliteEdge's leadership team and get the message out to agents, we were beginning to see results. We'd tried many different ideas to get the word out to agents that we offered a better health care option than is usually available to self-employed people. We'd tested numerous ways to communicate this value and get agents to engage with us, and it felt terrific to discover what worked. Executives were enthusiastic and supportive, which always helps. The presentations I did in scores of team meetings generated hundreds of appointments booked with our consultants. Webinars were also a big hit and also filled up the calendars. We were starting to reap the harvest from all of my efforts and that was incredibly satisfying!

Experiencing progress after hard work feels great, especially after the blows I'd suffered. I love the relationship between the level of exertion and length of time I exert to the depth of satisfaction I feel with the progress I made. Hard work that pays off is addicting. I definitely get dopamine hits for even tiny successes—which is magnified when the progress has direct and positive impact on people's lives and our own growth. This is my favorite formula on earth: Solving a big problem for others + collaboration and hard work = everyone wins!

After the wobble in 2020 during quarantine, EliteEdge grew so fast it was dizzying. It reminded me of my heady days at Dell in 1997, when I managed the website and we were the e-commerce darlings who were blazing new trails. I love the energy of rapidly traveling through unchartered territory and the excitement of helping companies solve big headaches for people in new ways. We were moving the needle. We were seeing results from our hard work, determination, and relentless but polite persistence. Once again, the consistent drum beat of persistence and expert relationship building was paying off big in my work. I'll take those wins!

It felt pretty easy to access gratitude for my work accomplishments. So, I focused on that satisfaction to grow my gratitude allowing myself to relish the success I'd earned while also helping others thrive. I also practiced a good amount of self-care. I felt grateful for my health and my deep and loving relationships. But the pandemic continued to roar on and by mid-February 2021, there were more than 27 million people in the U.S. with COVID. At the same exact time, I was cancer-free and I was having an incredibly successful year at work. Ain't that just like reality?

The irony about gratitude is it's so easy to come by when life is good; not so much when life lands a one-two punch that levels you. That's when you need them the most. I felt angry about the permanent changes to my body and I also felt deep grief over the three successive losses I'd faced. Plus, like 100 percent of the world, I was sick and tired of the freaking pandemic. I experienced days where I teetered on the edge of self-pity and sorrow. It was exhausting. However, I was able to appreciate that I could choose what I focused on, at least some of the time. And that meant I could feel gratitude—however small it may have been—for what was good and practice self-compassion when I didn't do a good job of choosing the happy feelings. This was a *hard* time. But at least I wasn't stuck in the feelings of anger, grief, and frustration all the time.

And just when I thought things were beginning to look up, shit got real... *again.*

***

No global pandemic would be complete without a major weather event to cripple an entire state. Much of Texas' electrical grid is above ground with lines running through the trees, leaving them vulnerable. Also, the heavy sleet that deluged on February 12, 2021, covered trees and power lines in ice and contributed to the power failures across the state.

We heard a loud creaking in the front yard and we saw a huge branch from our live oak crash onto the ground. We could hear this happening across the neighborhood. Our electricity went out later that afternoon. We had no way to cook, light, or heat our home. It was 28 degrees. Neat.

By nightfall, we broke out the battery-operated camping lantern and flashlights to help us see where we were going. We loaded Read and the dogs into the SUV and ventured out to find somewhere open where we could get food. As we drove very carefully, we saw dozens of flashes of red and green lights on the horizon. We lost count and wondered what we were seeing. Transformers going out? Turns out, yes! It looked like a bizarre red and green fireworks show low on the horizon. The ice was taking out the transformers and the entire electric grid of Texas was in danger of going down completely. We would later learn Texas is the only state in the U.S. that doesn't connect to other electrical grids—and it was a mess.

We hunkered down with a ton of blankets and made it through the night. It was 50 degrees inside, so weren't in danger of freezing to death, but that's not a very comfortable inside temperature. The storm dropped eight inches of the beautiful white stuff across the Austin area. It was treacherously beautiful. We kept hoping electricity would come on, but it didn't. The food in the refrigerator was going to spoil, so I, along with many other Texans, moved the groceries outdoors into coolers in the snow. It worked great! People sat in their cars to charge their phones and get warm.

The next day, our water went out. Of course we had no idea when that would come on, but it wasn't the next day. Or the next. Or even the next. After four days, the electricity came back on, but no water. My husband and I set up a snow collecting, melting, and straining station. We took storage bins out to the front yard and scooped up snow and the ice that was beneath it. My husband brought those full bins inside where we transferred the snow into a giant lobster pot on the stove. As snow and ice melted, we poured the water through a strainer to remove sticks, grass and dirt. This water was then taken to the tub closest to the kitchen. We kept a cooking pot near the fridge and used it to pour the water from the tub into the toilet so we could flush. Very *Little House on the Prairie.* Truth be told, it was fun, like an adventure. For the first day.

But as the waterless days dragged on, the three humans in our home started getting ripe. We were eager to have a warm shower! We found a hotel in San Antonio that allowed dogs and was on the same grid as a hospital, so we knew they would have electricity. I called to verify that they had electricity *and* hot water. They assured me they did, so we piled into the SUV—three adults and two large dogs—along with a week's worth of laundry and whatever groceries we had left. We were referred to as refugees from Austin and were grateful we could drive an hour and a half south and find warm accommodations. Of all the notable showers in my life—the first being the one I took following my cystectomy—this one ranked a close second.

The Texas power outage was hard on a lot of people beyond what we endured. People all over the state suffered worse. I acknowledge that yes, it was a rough (and somewhat smelly) time, but I was grateful we had the will and means to seek out small comforts, like a hot shower a short drive away, to help us weather this current storm (literally).

***

The 2021 Texas "snowpocalypse" that followed the endless suffering of 2020 very well could have been the straw that broke this camel's back. For me (and many others I'm sure), 2020 was one of the hardest years of my life. It's just that COVID-19 wasn't in my top three hard things that year. I had no idea how I was going to get through one day to the next. The pandemic had robbed us of many priceless experiences, including saying goodbye to our parents before they died. I could be bitter—and by all accounts I should be—but I'm not.

How did I make it through that valley of fear, fighting for my life and facing incredible losses? One second at a time. Thank goodness that I'd learned how to give myself compassion when I needed it! I certainly did not feel like doing anything, so I allowed myself some time to rest physically and emotionally. That meant I took several "depression naps." When my nervous system is overrun with grief, my body wants to collapse and sleep. It's the one time I can think of when it's easy for me to fall asleep. I felt as if I had no choice but to give into the emotional exhaustion. I gave myself compassion and permission to feel what I felt. I desperately wanted to feel anything but overwhelming grief, yet I knew that the quickest path to healing was straight through the middle—feeling it all and letting it happen. I couldn't have stopped it if I'd tried.

Thank goodness for the incredible love and devotion my husband gives me. And for the compassion and love I feel from my children, family and friends. Just as Coleman held me as I grieved my mother's death, I held and comforted him as he grieved his father's death just a few short months later. At least we did—and still do—have each other! To quote Bon Jovi, "and that's a lot of love!"

I know I'm repeating myself when I say how grateful I am for my husband, my family, and my friends. They are my "why" and what propelled me to keep going when I didn't feel like I could take another step. We all need to know our "whys" and be grateful for the time we have with them. What matters most to each of us varies. Understanding our deepest wants at the core of who we are empowers us to grasp onto whatever we're grateful for to keep us going when we feel like we can't take another step.

PART 3:

Healing and Rebounding

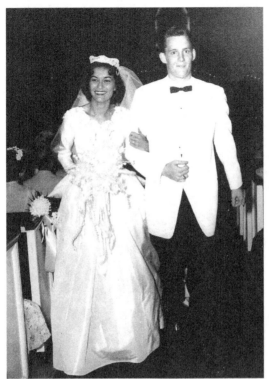
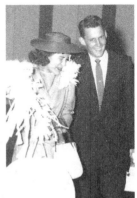
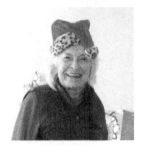
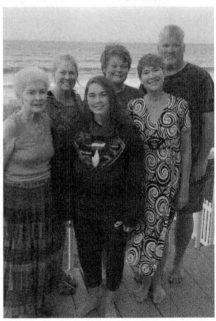
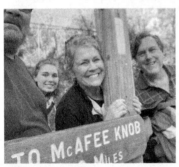
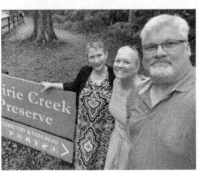

Chapter 12:
Looking Back to Forge Ahead

I could never have survived 2020's incessant stream of vicious blows without four things— healthy and loving relationships, gratitude, self-compassion, and learning from mistakes (mine and those of others). I collected these tools during the course of my life as I overcame some severe difficulties. Looking back on the lessons I learned from my parents, both good and bad, shows me the way forward—how to get back up time after time, blow after blow, when I didn't have another ounce of energy to fight. There were many times when just a tiny shard of gratitude and hope kept me moving forward.

Nurture Healthy Relationships

Growing healthy relationships is a lot like gardening: you plant seeds with care, provide nurturing love, pull weeds and prune when necessary, and ultimately enjoy the fruits born of your labor. I'm actually terrible gardener but I'm a really excellent relationship nurturer. I think it's because I am an extrovert who is energized by spending time with people and enjoying happy relationships. And the company of plants just doesn't do the same thing for me. No offense to all the passionate gardeners out there. As my daughter noticed how I communicate that I don't care for an activity, "It's not my thing."

One easy example I can think of for what nurturing a relationship means is staying in touch with people. And not just when I want something from them. Communicate by calling, texting, emailing, writing a note—whatever that person prefers. Let's use a totally and not-at-all real life example of an uncle who means a lot to you and has been very generous with his condo in Florida. In this hypothetical scenario, you love this uncle and enjoy spending time with him. He's funny and cool and has great stories. Of course you appreciate that he invites you to stay in his condo, but what you want to communicate to him is that your relationship with him is more valuable than a week in that sweet three-bedroom waterfront condo.

Let's imagine you're that uncle (or aunt or friend). Which would tell you that the family member values your relationship more important than the generous amenities you have to bestow?

A. An annual text saying you're planning a trip to Florida and asking if the condo is available.

B. The above annual text plus birthday and holiday texts.

C. All of the above and regular phone calls to catch up, hear stories, share a laugh, and enjoy time together.

D. None of the above. Wait for him to text or call.

C is correct! It's pretty straightforward to see some frequency of showing interest in people you care about is a good way to nurture the relationship. This is where being mindful with your intentions is key. When you see something that reminds you of this uncle or aunt, take a picture and send a text or call. Don't let that opportunity pass without making a point to show this person they are meaningful to you and you think about them. This is like feeding and watering plants in a garden. It's not going to happen without awareness and action. You can use the same principle for caring for personal relationships.

It's not hard and it's not time consuming, although it can take a bit more awareness. If you already do this, that's awesome! If not, you can absolutely learn how. Most of us want to be the thoughtful caring person and not *that* person who only reaches out when they want something.

Let's look at another opportunity for nurturing relationships. You've probably heard about the value of active listening. Have you ever been in a conversation with someone who was a chatty Cathy? Just one word after another, leaving you no opportunity to jump in and contribute one single sentence? Frustrating, isn't it? Also pretty boring. Even if you're not practicing active listening, the super talkative person might have even said, "You're such a good conversationalist!"

Contrast that experience with one where you've done the talking for a bit and the listener nods, reflects back what you've said and asks you questions. "You've just gotten certified to scuba dive? That sounds cool! Where do you want to go diving first?" Let's look at a more pedestrian topic. "You just started a new job selling health insurance? What are your plans for getting starting in this field? Where do you see the most interesting opportunities? What drew you into this industry?"

Humans want to feel heard and understood. So much so that when we feel heard, we feel more relaxed, more confident, better about ourselves. Actively listening to people is one of the greatest gifts you can give someone! It is also the foundation of relationship building.

Combatting the loneliness, pain, and fear of death during my cancer battle was one of the hardest struggles of my life. I relied on the strength of my relationships to provide the strength I lacked in order to keep going. With the isolation caused by the pandemic during my treatment, accessing the feelings of love and support from friends and family required more effort. I knew they were there for me, so I often closed my eyes and imagined them in the room with me, stroking my forehead, showering me with love, support, and encouragement. This helped me connect the cold and lonely present with warm and loving connections I knew were there in spirit. The loving bond I shared with my family and friends was a gift that I could appreciate. It was also a gift that gave me enough strength to survive this unimaginable journey, so I could enjoy thriving again.

Gratitude with Gritted Teeth

I'd recognized in high school that feeling optimistic felt better than feeling sorry for myself. So I was partway to embracing gratitude. Eager to keep feeling happy and hopeful, I continued learning and playing the Grateful Game to grow my practice of gratitude.

Focusing on what was good in my life was how I got through this challenging year and other dark times I've experienced. The relationships with those I loved were what I treasured most. They were my "why." When I felt like giving up—and I did feel like giving up, often—I dug deep and persevered through those hard times by thinking about the people I loved and who loved me.

Gratitude is very interesting. Studies conducted on how our brains react when we are focusing on feeling grateful reveal some fascinating data. No matter how small the item is that is the focus of appreciation, our brains respond very positively. They send signals to produce the happy hormones and refrain from sending signals to produce stress hormones such as cortisol.

That means focusing on our own gratitude can change the chemistry in our brains! It's not just a woo-woo platitude. Appreciating what we can about our lives makes us feel happier. That seems like an amazing life hack! Plus, zero calories and fat, costs nothing, hurts no one, and will likely help several people. *Score!*

Sometimes, I felt so overwhelmed by grief that it seemed impossible to think of anything I could appreciate. My therapist helped me see that I was grieving the loss of how I looked, not just to me, but also to the outside world. Chemo does not improve one's skin tone, hairstyle, energy level, or fingernails. A radical cystectomy does not improve a woman's figure. This is exacerbated by nature's gifts to women during menopause. Weight seems to move around and not in an owner-of-the-body directed way. I did not approve my body to shift weight from my butt to my waist, even though I hadn't gained weight. My waistline just seemed to expand, while my curves seemed to evaporate. Super cool. And now, I had extra bulk in exactly the one place I wanted to shrink. I was *so* mad! I still am sometimes. It's hard to feel attractive when you look in the mirror and see a bald, barrel-shaped version of yourself with a big ol' plastic bag stuck to your waist.

Now, is this the most important thing for me to dwell upon? No. Does it mean that my feelings of disappointment, frustration, and loss are invalid? Also no. With the help from the Bladder Cancer Advocacy Network, support groups, my therapist, friends, and my loving husband, I learned to accept how I felt and also to acknowledge the things I appreciated, such as the rockstar medical professionals at MD Anderson who saved my freaking life!

And man, that is some hard work! It's exhausting to feel the negative feelings and acknowledge overwhelming anger and sadness. I can certainly see why stuffing or numbing those emotions is an easy choice to make, whether an intentional choice or not. Bummer that Brené Brown is right about numbing. We can't select specific areas to numb as if we're injecting Novocaine specifically to one area. Nope, the numbing is universal, which means the distractions we use to minimize our pain also minimize our joy. So much for peanut M&M's as my primary numbing agent.

***

It's a strange feeling to face death. For my whole life up until this point, I was afraid of dying. My beliefs about what happens after we die can best be described as a colorful and non-linear journey.

I was raised garden-variety Christian in the deep south. We were members of a Methodist church and like most families we knew, we went to church and Sunday school most weeks. My parents sang in the choir and when I was about 13, I joined MYF, the Methodist Youth Group. That was fun, because we hung out with friends and our youth leader who was a surfer dude with shoulder-length blonde hair—which was pretty rad in 1975! Ironically, MYF was where I was first exposed to marijuana, which was still very illegal back then. It's not my thing.

My parents taught us to think for ourselves. I remember being about 11 years old and having what might have been my first deeply profound thought. I asked my parents, "How could Adam and Eve been the first people on earth a few thousand years ago when we descended from primates over the course of millions of years?" Now remember, this was in the early 1970s and evolution was just gaining credibility and being introduced to school curriculum. Also, how did Adam and Eve populate the earth with people when they had two sons and one of them killed the other one? There had to be some more people somewhere.

I still remember how they answered. They offered the possibility that perhaps Adam and Eve were the first humans given names. My brain lit up thinking about that. When did we begin verbally communicating? When did we start giving ourselves names? When did we first create a written language? When did we learn to control fire?

I believed in God and heaven and enjoyed the parental and church support of questioning and seeking answers. If you weren't a murderer or a rapist and you tried your best to be a good person, then going to heaven after death was ensured. Over the next decades, I would wander in and out of churches and the details of my faith were somewhat fluid. I never felt that angry God thing. Protestants are focused much more on the New Testament, which takes place after God took some anger management courses. Lord, I apologize about that.

By the time I hit my 50s, I was feeling more aligned with a broad belief in a connected universe, about which we understand very little, and which is utterly fascinating. The mammoth scientific discoveries that continued to occur delivered more questions than answers. Like when we thought we understood that the universe is made of matter, and we discovered that some of the matter was dark matter. And later we discovered anti-matter, which is mind blowing to me. I can completely understand how every culture has created some belief system or religion to explain what they couldn't possibly understand.

I didn't know if heaven was a real place or an allegory of the peace and beauty that appears to our souls when we die. I have no idea what happens when we die, and I prefer believing that we go to heaven and get to see our loved ones who've gone before us. As I lay in bed after each round of chemo, feeling miserable and nauseated, in pain with a splitting headache and ringing in my ears, I thought, "If I died, I wouldn't personally feel sad, because I'd just be gone and no longer aware or possibly better off in a wonderful afterlife." Once I saw my own mortality this way, my fear of death evaporated and my gratitude blossomed. Strange but also positive.

With fear out of the way, I found it so much easier to feel newly grateful for things I took for granted before. Clean drinking water, a safe and comfortable place to live, friends I adore, a husband and family I love more than life itself, two eyes that give me sight to take in the beauty in the world. The flood gates of gratitude were open all the way! It felt amazing!

Doing harm to myself never crossed my mind, fortunately. I did experience some peace when that fear of my life ending evaporated. The chemo treatment was just so miserable to experience and my brain was so foggy that I did have moments when I felt like my end could be near, and I accepted that. Also, we didn't know if all this treatment and surgery would be successful and that was a whole other surreal burden to bear! So many existential lessons at one time.

Self-Compassion

Self-compassion was a relatively new concept to me. I found it incredibly freeing to have permission to go easy on myself! You mean, it's okay to be nice to myself and change my inner dialogue to one that's loving and supportive? This was an amazing addition to my suite of coping skills!

Facing so much grief offered me far too many opportunities to practice self-compassion. Trying this out on myself was a brand-new experience. I don't think I'd ever heard the term until several years before, and I certainly had no experience *actually practicing* it. Reading Dr. Kristen Neff's book, *Fierce Self-Compassion: How Women Can Harness Kindness to Speak Up, Claim Their Power, and Thrive,* was eye-opening! Being kind to myself was as foreign of a concept as time travel.

I worried that practicing self-compassion would be indulgent and counterproductive. There's that Calvinistic work ethic shining through. I like my work ethic and enjoy getting things done and the achievements of my efforts. It feels great, is socially acceptable, and was highly praised in my family of origin. It's also super handy for succeeding in work and life.

But was working, task completion, and accomplishing my numbing agent? (Sharp intake of breath. *M-a-y-b-e?*) That was a terrifying potential realization! I can stop anytime. I don't have to finish one more thing before I close the computer for the night...

"Hello, my name is Margo and I'm a workaholic. It's been none minutes since I last worked to complete a task."

"Hi, Margo."

Because I wanted to try self-compassion, I decided to refrain from labeling myself as anything, especially anything -*aholic*. I thought it could be interesting to test this self-compassion concept. It sounded lovely if a bit uncomfortable. Being kind to myself felt awkward at first, even though this wasn't a for-the-public's-viewing experience. Beating myself up was a lot more familiar, since I had 50-something years practice at it. Negative self-talk was familiar but extremely unpleasant. I was ready for a more pleasant experience. I felt comforted knowing I wasn't alone.

In her book, Dr. Neff defines the three elements of self-compassion as self-kindness vs. self-judgment, common humanity vs. isolation, mindfulness vs. overidentification. The self-kindness vs. self-judgment lesson nearly broke my brain. I didn't fully understand how strong the role of self-talk was in my life until I was in my 30s. One of my favorite therapists observed that I might be verbally abusive to myself. I was shocked and a bit horrified to hear that and realize it might be true. I never set out to be mean to myself. Self-talk comes from deep within our consciousness, which is why recognizing its impact is so helpful. Most of the messages we receive every day are from our own minds, and most are negative! Which is actually pretty convenient because those are the only ones we can impact.

I've learned to speak kindly to myself when I'm feeling grumpy or not-so-grateful. Years of therapy and soaking up wisdom from others has taught me that self-compassion is healthy. I was raised by people descended from Quakers and hard work is our love language. Suffering from working hard and helping others showed that you met the minimum level of criteria required for acceptance. Speaking highly of yourself was seen as boastful, even sinful. Ergo, negative self-talk had an environment ripe for growing strong.

Not that controlling our inner dialogue is easy. It is not; however it *is* possible. And that is so freeing! We have so many resources available to help us with this. Journaling is especially helpful to me. One of my favorite ways to start my day is with a cup of strong coffee, my journal, and making a list of 10 things for which I am grateful. Sometimes that list includes very small or basic things, like clean water to drink, food to eat, a safe home to live in, a body that is strong, ears so I can hear the cicadas and the birds in the morning. I invite you to try it and let me know how it goes for you.

What worked for me was thinking about Dr. Neff's suggestion of treating ourselves with the same kindness that we treat others with. They deserve love and I deserve love. We are all worthy of love and acceptance! I felt like a weight had been lifted off my shoulders. How freeing to know that I can treat myself with the love and respect I want and deserve. And that it feels good to treat myself that way. Thinking about how I talk with the people I care most about helped me know what to say to myself. Reflecting on how they talked to and encouraged me also helped. I felt supported and cared for and loved. And somehow this exercise surprised me. Why wouldn't saying the same things to myself that I say to people I love *not* feel good?

The common humanity part of self-compassion is very powerful. Something about our experiences being shared is comforting. I think it's because we have evolved to live in community with each other and shared experiences is a key component of it all. We yearn to relate to each other, share experiences, and help each other endure. Ultimately, we share a desire to enjoy life and share warm, positive, and beautiful experiences together.

Understanding the common humanity connection—that I share many of these challenges and feelings with my human sisters and brothers—made trying out some self-compassion a little easier. I wanted to feel better about myself and apparently, I wasn't alone. So, I took self-compassion out for a spin and it went pretty well. Even though it felt strange to talk to myself in comforting ways, I noticed that I felt better once I accepted encouraging talk from my own head. I can't imagine how it could hurt. I've read that talking to ourselves in the third person is more effective, so I do that sometimes. LeBron James does this and his track record speaks for itself.[14]

---

14 Amy Morin, *Friday Fix: Why Lebron James Talks to Himself in the Third Person* (and Why You Should Too), podcast, https://www.verywellmind.com/friday-fix-why-lebron-james-talks-to-himself-in-the-third-person-and-why-you-should-too-5185654.

So, it's effective, simple, and free? Sign me up. I continued to read Dr. Neff's books and enrolled in one of her online courses. I learned so much from that experience and highly recommend her work.[15] And be kind to yourself as you explore this new journey of practicing self-compassion. As you may have guessed, it's not a linear journey. However, the benefits are outstanding.

Learn from Your Mistakes and the Mistakes of Others

These are the hardest lessons I learned from my parents and from my own life—admitting mistakes and learning from the mistakes of others. Some of these ended up being gifts as well, just not very pleasant ones to learn. Learning from mistakes is a lifelong journey.

Paying attention to what felt good about how my mother and father raised me gave me a great list of what to do to raise healthy children. Noticing how bad I felt when my own parents failed to do their best for me provided me with a list what not to do for raising my own kids.

Anger isn't empowering. The marriage between my two smart, hurt, and defensive parents went as you might expect it would go. They fought a lot. They both yelled, screamed, and threw and broke things in anger. They also said very mean things to all of us when they raged. They didn't apologize later and I hated the way that felt. If parents don't apologize for hurting kids emotionally or physically, the children internalize the pain as earned, deserved. I made a mental note to myself: When I'm a mother, do not say mean things and shout at my kids. And if I do get mad and lose my temper, apologize to them right away.

It's scary growing up with that amount of turmoil and rage. Although my parents never drank, they had many behaviors and coping skills that I later learned were characteristic of alcoholics. They were rage-aholics and never realized it. My siblings and I thought this was normal, as kids are prone to think of their own childhood experiences. Because parents are humans and humans are imperfect, parenting perfectly rarely, if ever occurs. I came to

---

15 Check out Dr. Neff's website to find what appeals most to you: https://self-compassion.org/store/.

realize that my parents were doing the best they could and sometimes that wasn't very good.

Losing our temper was almost encouraged in my family of origin. That makes sense for a household headed by ragers. So, yes, I try not to lose my temper, and also I'm wired with a shorter fuse than I'd like. My mom seemed to channel her empowerment through her anger and after a while, I began to feel like that was twisted and distorted. I remember stomping on an etch-a-sketch as a 14-year-old and feeling terrible about it! I cried and told my parents how bad I felt and they were understanding and didn't punish me. I'm glad they didn't, since that would have compounded things, but I thought they might want to give me some guidance on taming my temper. They couldn't.

After years of therapy, I learned that anger is not, in fact, all that empowering. Anger is an important emotion to acknowledge and experience, but we don't need to celebrate it, act on it, or encourage its dysfunction.

Most people aren't out to get me. My mother seemed to view the world through "People are out to do me wrong" lenses, which was sad. And she was very up front about how angry she felt about being treated poorly. I remember her being angry a lot. Her keen mind was well trained at observation and critical thinking, which resulted in me feeling criticized and "not enough." I'm pretty sure I'm not alone in feeling this way. Imposter syndrome is real.

I recall sharing concerns with my mom that I had about whether I'd get invited to a birthday party when I was in the seventh grade. She was very sympathetic, but something didn't feel right. Her response was concern for me, yes. But I felt like she almost got energized by my feeling left out. She held me and tried to sooth me, but I was wanting encouragement for how to engage with the friends more so I would get invited and she was focused on how unfair it was. I wanted to change it, not accept the social failure! We had different goals for this conversation. I didn't like how that felt either, so I decided to edit what I shared with her in the future, in order to take care of myself and to keep my relationship with my mother as healthy as it could be. I didn't know it at the time, but this was healthy self-care and it felt right. I was beginning to understand where to establish boundaries for keeping my relationship with my mother okay for me.

Respect other people's boundaries. And while we're talking about boundaries, just like good fences make good neighbors, healthy boundaries support healthy relationships.

One memory that stands out is when I was 12 and came home from school tired. I was attending public school, which was a sixth-grade center in a very poor neighborhood. The school was rough, and the kids were rougher. I didn't have many friends or feel comfortable there, so I had some unpleasant experiences at school. Although I really loved my teacher and the one-day-a-week gifted program where she taught evolution, dinosaurs, plate tectonics, and the frightening novels by Edgar Allan Poe— this particular day was not one of those days and I was spent.

I plopped down on the sofa and my mom asked, "What's wrong?" I replied, "I'm just tired." "It seems like more than that," she prodded. I told her I was really just tired from school. But she kept digging, which began to annoy me. I thought to myself, "Geesh, Mom, just let me be! I'm just tired and would like you to stop asking me a bunch of times if there's more to it than that." This may seem minor or even petty. What I didn't understand then was that I was attempting to set a boundary for my comfort level with this conversation and she was not respecting that boundary. And I didn't like how that felt at all.

This was a pattern with my mom. I understood even then that she did love me and wanted to help me. And I also understood it was okay for me to have boundaries and it was not okay that she didn't respect them.

Don't overstay your welcome. The dysfunction, anger, and turmoil in our home were at a fever pitch by the summer I graduated high school. My father had moved out and was divorcing my mother. I couldn't *wait* to get to college and start *my* life without them! I had fallen in love with UNC Chapel Hill, and became the second generation of women in my family to attend. My mom drove me to North Carolina to move me into my dorm. That part went fine.

I could see that my mother felt sad to leave her oldest daughter at college several states away while she was going through a divorce. What wasn't fine was when she asked to stay in my dorm room with me that first night, since my roommate hadn't shown up. What could I say? I felt sorry for her and didn't feel like I had the right to say "no" and make her feel bad. She'd taught me to feel responsible for her happiness. *And that is not okay.* But I didn't know that then.

That first night the college held a freshman welcome party. It was so much fun! We all wore white t-shirts and wrote on each other's shirts with magic markers. Loud 80's music boomed loudly while lights flashed and 18-year-olds had a lot of fun. "Everybody Wang Chung" and "Super Freak" stand out as fun memories of that night. But I also have the memory that my mom came to the party. She was cool but I was the only freshman with a parent at the party. I had such a great time but it was really *weird* to have her there. I loved her but also really wanted her to leave. My mother finally left the next day, and I knew she was sad and lonely. I felt bad for her and wanted to make things better for her, but I couldn't.

I made another note to myself: Do not overstay your welcome when you take your kids to college. And when it was my turn, I didn't.

Do not make my kids feel responsible for my happiness. It would be many years of me over-functioning and trying to meet the goal of being "enough" for my mom before I would realize there would never be enough. It was a trick. Her need for emotional support was a black hole. It wasn't her intent. I know she loved me. And also, she was a taker.

I remember being eight months pregnant with my first child and flying to Tampa for a baby shower that my friends threw for me. My mother still lived in Jacksonville, and I allowed her to make me feel guilty for going to Tampa without coming to see her, so I altered my plans and took another couple of days to fly into Jacksonville and spend some time with her. I was working at Dell with a senior level job, so my time was tightly scheduled and making this change was a big deal for me to do.

When it was time for me to drive to Tampa, she complained about me leaving her. "Don't your friends realize that I need you more than they do?"

I responded through tears, "I'm not going because they need me, I'm going because they love me and want to celebrate with me that I'm having a baby." And I wished so much that she could stop putting her needs ahead of mine. I cried all the way to Tampa and was so happy to see my friends and start laughing and celebrating.

I made yet another note to myself: Do not make your kids feel responsible for your happiness.

Do not be guilted by the insecurities of others. I distinctly remember my mom asking me why I wanted to spend time with my friends. *Um, because I'm extroverted and that's normal?* I felt like an alien, born of these two introverted and angry people.

I called Atlanta home for two years. When I'd visit Florida, my mother would guilt me into not seeing friends. Yes, I know now that I allowed her to do that. But displeasing her didn't feel like a viable option then. So, I visited Jacksonville as infrequently as possible and never moved back there. I did not want more drama, negativity, and rage in my life, but I felt guilty if I didn't visit my mother. One of the harder lessons I learned was how to set and enforce boundaries with my mom. My mom also was judgmental and disapproving of my mate choices. She wasn't wrong about some of them, but yelling at me wasn't the way to help me see that. It was all so difficult and confusing. And let's face it—we want to be accepted and loved by our parents. Setting boundaries with some parents, like my mother, put that love and acceptance at risk. Those are high stakes and I had no experience with it at all.

Using trial and error over the course of decades, I struggled with this delicate balance of boundaries, self-care, and my role as a daughter. My mother wanted my time in Jacksonville all to herself and of course, I wanted to please her and have her love me. So, I did not contact my old friends from high school. Instead, I allowed relationships I valued to be sacrificed to please my mom. She wanted me to stay longer, never see my dad, and avoid seeing friends. I wanted to be "enough" for her to love me. But it was never enough.

Now, I understand that no amount of sacrifice is enough to earn complete acceptance and unconditional love from someone who is very selfish, narcissistic, or insecure. And it doesn't matter how sad the story is of how these people came to be so selfish. The net result is that it's impossible to ever be enough for people who primarily think of themselves. Even if those people are your parents. This was such a hard lesson for me to learn and I know I'm not the only one learning it because so many people have shared similar stories with me.

Here's the hope I want to share with you about navigating through the difficult waters of relationships with selfish or narcissistic people: It's absolutely possible to break out of the bondage of attempting and always failing to be enough for them. We deserve acceptance, love, and caring. Sometimes, our parents or other people in our lives do not have the capacity to give us those things. So give the gifts of acceptance, love, and caring to yourself!

Self-care is not selfish. No matter what the self-centered person says. Parents who manipulate their children into denying healthy choices for themselves are acting only out of self-interest. Taking care of yourself is not only healthy and worth setting boundaries, it's how you take back the reigns of your emotional and physical well-being.

All this ridiculous guilt helped me learn this lesson: Accept and love my kids for who they are and prioritize our close relationship above all else. One of the keys to nurturing a close relationship with kids is to give them room to enjoy other relationships. This allows them to feel safe to maintain a healthy balance of taking care of their own needs and not take responsibility for making their parents happy.

Do not make a crisis about me. After the death of my kids' father, my mom—who had declined my multiple offers to fly her to Texas for a visit—said, "My grandchildren need me to help them grieve the loss of their father." No, they don't. She'd barely been in their lives and she'd criticized them during the few times she had been. She just wanted to insert herself into our current disaster because it released adrenaline in her brain. My sweet boyfriend at the time, Coleman, sat beside me as I had this awkward phone call. He helped me craft a response and enforce my boundary with her: "I appreciate that Mom, and I am declining your offer. I'm comfortable with how we're moving through this right now."

***

I believe these lessons I learned throughout my life have been invaluable in establishing healthy relationships and boundaries with my own children and in my other relationships—and also with myself. Focusing on gratitude, self-care, self-compassion, and the other positive aspects in my life have released me from the anger and dysfunction that bound me as I grew up, and prepared me with coping mechanisms for future challenges. It's a conscious and willing choice I gladly make every day.

Conclusion:
When Enough Is Just Enough

How do we persist when we don't feel like it or when we are exhausted? It's a relief to know we don't have to 100 percent *feel* like going to keep going. Actually, we don't have to feel any percent like persevering. I think that's one of the beliefs that can get in our way. We don't need to feel motivated to take the next right step. The answer to the burning question of how to keep going when we lack the drive or energy is to simply use whatever we have—and that's just enough to propel us forward.

One of my favorite examples is when I'm tired and don't feel like exercising. Of course, I know it's good for my body, mind, and soul to get outside and move around. But there are times when I just don't feel like it. At all. So I acknowledge that I don't feel like it and give myself some self-compassion. I have a little conversation with myself, "I know. You're tired, you had a long day, work is stressful, and the last thing you want to do is walk around in this Texas heat and get sweaty. I get it. You know what? You don't have to go for a long walk or even a short one. No expectations. Just put on your shoes and stand up, okay? Maybe take a couple of steps toward the door and then step outside." Most of the time I'm walking before I know it. And sure, I may not set any cardio records, but a short bit of exercise is better than no exercise. Plus, there's a side benefit: I feel a little bit better about myself and my mood is little better!

This works for a few reasons. First, this approach removes the pressure to have my mindset or attitude adjusted before I can take action. In fact, there is zero requirement for me to feel motivated. I can feel as unmotivated as I want and that's not a problem.

Second, I've reduced the goal down to nano-sized. Instead of setting a goal of having to walk 30 minutes or 10 or even one minute, I've broken it down to just putting shoes on. The smallest unit of taking action to go for a walk I can think of. Putting shoes on doesn't require any motivation, determination, or drive. It's like breathing. Just put them on and see what happens.

Third, having no expectations takes all the pressure and judgement off me. Doesn't matter if I even make it outside, just see what happens. Just observe. That's it. Removing expectations and judgment of how I'm doing against those expectations removes the friction to taking action. So, there's no risk I'm going to feel bad for underperforming. Okay, so I really can't lose here. That's pretty cool.

Finally, this ends up being an act of self-compassion. By treating myself like I would a friend or loved one, I'm giving love and support to me at a time when I really need it. Accepting where I am in this moment and simply noticing how I'm feeling is incredibly nurturing. Removing all expectations and performance goals is freeing and courageous.

Courage isn't the absence of fear: it's taking action in the face of fear. That's all I could do—through cancer and loss and grief—and it was enough. It didn't feel good, but it was enough. I most certainly did not feel like staying in the hospital for several nights. I was uncomfortable, exhausted, lonely, and fed up with the incessant pokes and prods! If I'd felt any better, I might have been tempted to run screaming down the hall to escape. But I could barely walk around the nurse's station, so that wasn't a risk. I desperately wanted to get out of there and be home with my husband and family.

How did I get through those long and lonely days and night? One minute at a time. Sometimes I would focus on my breathing and count my breaths. Sometimes I would think about happy experiences, like my honeymoon in Grand Cayman just three-and-a-half years earlier. Sometimes I tried to watch a funny movie. And sometimes I had to muster every bit of self-compassion I could think of and give myself a little pep-talk: "I know this is impossibly hard, Margo. You've already been through so much! This isn't fair and you understand that. You are loved and you are cherished by your sweet husband, wonderful children, and amazing friends and family. Focus on your gratitude for them. *They* need you and even if you don't *feel* like fighting this disease another minute, *you can and you will,* one reluctant, painstaking, nano-step at a time. You are doing the best you can and that is good enough!"

I want you to feel hopeful that you can also get through the hardest of times, the darkest of challenges. Even when you feel like giving up. It's okay to feel like giving up! It's okay to admit you don't have a tiny ounce of motivation to keep moving. Not only is all of this okay, it's actually healthy! Acknowledge how you really feel. Even it it's overwhelmed and hopeless. The secret I want to share with you is that you can keep going, even when you are completely out of motivation. All you have to do is not die, to keep fighting. And I know you can and you will do that!

Because enough is all you'll ever need.

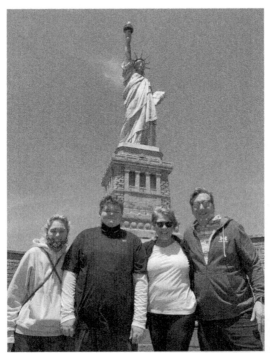
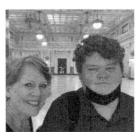
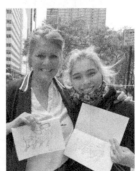
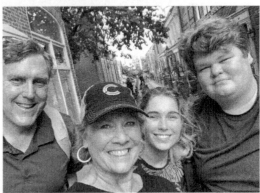
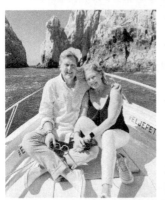
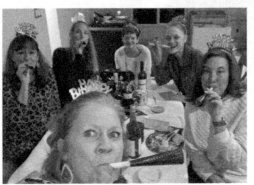
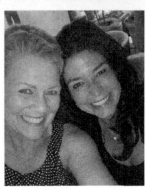

Afterword

Celebrating after enduring a life-or-death crisis and multiple deaths of loved ones during a global pandemic was on the menu for my family and me. Remembering and fully embracing the "Celebrate the Important Moments in Life" lesson, I planned a very special trip for our family to acknowledge Read's college graduation. We'd all experienced so many hard knocks and losses that a family trip seemed like a great way to celebrate not only Read's accomplishment, but also our collective triumph over the worst year we'd ever experienced. Read could choose to go anywhere in the U.S., and he picked NYC. Although we were all vaccinated, the idea of traveling internationally was daunting and the rest of the world wasn't fully open again yet. We all understood there was a risk that the pandemic could derail our trip, but we planned as if it wouldn't.

And there was planning, planning, planning! New York had been hit very hard and early in the pandemic and had been in an extended lockdown. Videos of empty streets were simply surreal, as if the city that never sleeps were hibernating. I carefully researched New York's vaccine and travel requirements. Because we were coming from Texas—a state that had opened earlier in the pandemic and was one of the "hot spots" with a high occurrence of COVID infections—we had to meet specific travel requirements. It was difficult to find the details and understand exactly what we could and couldn't do amid fluid and ever-changing protocols.

I've never spent more time planning a trip! It was 10 times more complicated than any other trip, due to the reduced hours for attractions, reduced capacities, and increased pandemic requirements. I made a spreadsheet of everything we wanted to see and the days and hours they operated. By September 2020, New York City had reopened some indoor dining with a maximum capacity of just 25 percent. Many attractions were either closed or at 25 percent capacity as well. All Broadway shows had been cancelled since March 12, 2020, and didn't open until September 2021.

I asked each family member to provide several "must sees." I wished I had had an app to run the data to develop the ideal itinerary, but none existed that included pandemic planning. I also considered the varying interests and energy levels in our family. No way would we have time to see everything. The goal was to enjoy ourselves and see the sites that mattered to us. I built buffer time into each day's schedule, which ended up being a very smart thing to do!

This trip seemed almost charmed! The four of us got along beautifully. No one complained and we even laughed at each other's jokes! When they were younger, they often disagreed on destinations, much like any children. "Can we *please* go somewhere that serves something besides burgers, chicken tenders or pizza?" my daughter would beg. "I can't help that I'm picky," my son would reply. But this trip, there was none of that.

We had two rooms with city views at the Millennium Times Square. When we checked in on Sunday, Times Square was eerily empty with barely any people out and about. It was the strangest experience to see the Big Apple looking like the Big Empty. My kids asked me if this was normal and my husband and I both answered, *"No!"* It's usually wall-to-wall people with a lot of outrageous characters.

We saw many closed restaurants and far too many "Available for Lease" signs on retail store fronts. New York had been hit especially hard by the pandemic. The high concentration of people from all over the world made the spread of coronavirus explode in the urban centers. I felt sad for the business owners who had lost so much as a result of this awful pandemic. And I felt grateful that my husband and I had jobs that were continuing to grow and thrive.

Our trip was peppered with many unusual experiences due to then pandemic restrictions, starting with our first meal. When we asked the concierge for restaurant recommendations, her answer was so weird for NYC:

"All of the restaurants and food service are suspended at the hotel and many restaurants have closed. Of the ones that are still in business, very few are open Sundays." I almost felt like we were back in a small town in Texas, where they rolled up the sidewalk on Saturday night and remained closed until Monday. We settled for a mediocre Mediterranean diner that was open nearby. Our food wasn't very good and the service was terrible, but we remained hopeful that we'd find a great restaurant open somewhere in the city.

I'd made reservations to tour the Guggenheim, and I drank in the unique spiral architecture and interesting artwork, like I had during a high school trip. But instead of being busy like it usually would have been, it was oddly dark inside, not crowded, and some of the walls had no artwork at all on them.

I think our practice of managing our expectations helped us remain flexible and we enjoyed our trip better as a result. We all met at 9:00 am, early enough to have time to enjoy several experiences throughout the day but also late enough to get a good sleep. It helped that I pre-booked tickets for many of the main attractions. I planned no more than one museum per day to avoid museum burnout and built in some downtime for late in the afternoons.

We went full tourist by booking a Big Bus Tour for our first full day. We sat on the upper deck so we could have unobstructed views. We loved hearing the interesting history that the recording provided, like the fact that Jackie Kennedy Onassis was instrumental in preserving Grand Central Station, among other buildings. We also learned the Flat Iron building had the last hydraulic elevator remaining in NYC, which took 30 long minutes to reach the top and wasn't replaced until 1999. Hearing about the waves of immigrants coming to New York and living in crowded tenement housing was moving. We imagined how awful life must have been for them in their original country if immigrating to America only to share a tiny apartment with 10 family members was the better choice.

The Big Bus Tour was a fun way to discover which attractions were most appealing to us. The experience was exciting and we had such a good time together! After a year and a half of the pandemic and my cancer battle and family member deaths, it felt invigorating to get out and see the world with my family again. I'm reminded of Robert Earl Keen's lyrics, "It feels so good to feel good again."

The other highlights of our trip were the Metropolitan Museum of Art—my family had to remind me to keep moving because we could *never* see it all in one afternoon!—and the Morgan Library, which my son had chosen for us to visit. The architecture was truly stunning, and we each appreciated something different about our experience there.

For his special dinner to celebrate his graduation from college, Read requested a steak dinner at Peter Luger's. We couldn't wait to taste this famous steak. *It was delicious.* But once again, our service was lacking—I chalked it up to the pressures of the pandemic placing additional stress on the restaurant employees. I found it unfortunate that our waiter's curt and unhelpful attitude is a memory we made there, but we enjoyed the food very much anyway and I was pleased we'd been able to take our family to a place Read had always wanted to go.

But a marvelous thing emerged during our trip. Each evening, we noticed more people on the streets and in Times Square. A few days before we arrived, New York Governor Cuomo had announced increased capacity for outdoor and indoor restaurants and museums, bringing capacity up to 33 percent. We were watching New York open back up live, in real time. It was an amazing sight to see!

It reminded me of the scene in the *Wizard of Oz,* where the Munchkins very cautiously peered from behind buildings to see with their own eyes if the Wicked Witch of the East was truly dead. It felt that way to me, too, as if I were cautiously emerging from a year-long nightmare into a strange new world.

Life can forge ahead despite adversity. There's only one way to move, and that's forward—one miniscule, laborious step at a time, clutching every scrap of gratitude you can find. Because when it comes down to the heart of the matter, the least amount of gratitude is just enough to keep you fighting the good fight for another day.

Gratitudes

Thanks to my editor and champion, Phyllis Jask, who magically knew how to pull better sentences out of my head to make my first book better than I could imagine. I appreciate Brenda Hawkes for her creativity and vision for making this book look and feel perfect.

I'm grateful for the never-ending love, support, and encouragement of my friends: Suzanne Danuser, Mari Hawn, Juli Herren, Anita Johnson, Milana McLead, Anna McQuaid, Michele Melo, Helen Patterson, Kathi Scott, Nanci Tucker, Kim Anderson, Lori Wasserburger, and so many others. I graciously thank my therapists, who helped me get unstuck and out of my own way, Rita Thompson and Dr. Jenny Pelquen.

I lovingly thank my family for their love, support, and encouragement: my late mother, Susan Berry; my brother, Craig Wickersham; my sister, Karen Wickersham; my uncle, Gene McCutchin; my grandparents, Mama Mac and Daddy Mac; and the woman who is like my other mother, Cora Greene.

My gratitude for all of the caregivers who provided me with life-saving treatments is immense. So many people at MD Anderson provided warm, attentive, and respectful care to me throughout my many solo stays at the hospital.

To my employers, I share my gratitude for their compassion, encouragement, and flexibility throughout my battles.

With a grateful heart, I am donating a portion of my book sales to BCAN, the Bladder Cancer Advocacy Network. Learn more about how you can support bladder cancer research at https://bcan.org/.

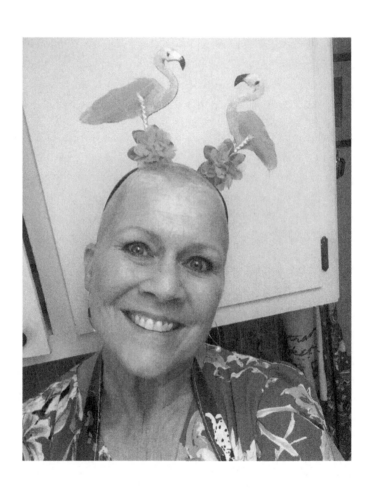

About the Author

The tenacious Margo Wickersham learned early in life that relationship building is her superpower, and she's exercised that skill throughout her life to help others help themselves. With relentless and fierce perseverance, she endured soul-crushing challenges, unbearable physical pain, and shocking emotional and bodily losses during a year that challenged the entire world. Her ability to channel gratitude strengthened her grit and determination beyond her wildest imagination, which she credits—along with the doctors at MD Anderson—for surviving and thriving after cancer and loss.

After surviving all that 2020 and 2021 threw at her, Margo adopted the mindset of saying yes to everything that makes life more enjoyable. This Florida native has always loved being by or in the water, so her most recent "yes" is a backyard pool—"the world's most expensive dog toy" in her husband's words. Margo has been saying yes to SCUBA diving since 1988.

She worked full-time to earn her degree in journalism from the University of North Carolina at Chapel Hill, and has enjoyed a varied and colorful sales and marketing career ever since. As a dell.com website manager, Margo led her team to create an award-winning redesign of the ecommerce site, created and launched successful PR and marketing campaigns, and built partner programs from the ground up. She is a licensed insurance agent, a licensed Realtor®, and an accomplished trainer, speaker, and writer. Margo has appeared in the *Wall Street Journal*, *Tampa Business Journal*, *West Austin News*, *Money Inc.*, *Self Esteem Magazine* and *Exceptional People Magazine*, among others. She has written blogs; participated as a guest on several podcasts and YouTube channels, including the Bladder

Cancer Awareness Network (BCAN) and MD Anderson Cancer Center; and been featured as a guest speaker at numerous local, national, and international events.

Well before self-publishing was commonplace, Margo published her grandparents' memoirs, an onerous yet rewarding task. As she presented the finished books to her grandparents while visiting them in Pensacola, Florida, a *Pensacola Times* reporter captured the touching moment and printed the story on the front cover of the *People* section.

The proud mother of Read and Rachel, Margo takes every opportunity to spend time with them and her wonderful husband Coleman. She and Coleman are thriving empty-nesters in Austin, Texas, where they walk and hike with their two dogs, Casey—a Lab and pool aficionado—and Nova—a Greyhound and landlubber.

Margo wants to hear your stories of gratitude, grit, and perseverance!

Connect with Margo on social media:

instagram.com/MargoWickersham

linkedin.com/in/MargoWickersham

facebook.com/MargoWickersham

twitter.com/MargoWickersham

tiktok.com/@MargoWickersham

bit.ly/MargoYoutube

Printed in Great Britain
by Amazon

11660550R00099